PATHOLOGY and MANAGEMENT of LYMPHOMA

edited by

John G. Allison, M.D.

Associate Professor of Surgery
Department of Surgery
Medical University of South Carolina;
Chief, Surgical Services
Veterans Administration Medical Center
Charleston, South Carolina

1984
Futura Publishing Company
Mount Kisco, New York

Published by
Futura Publishing Company, Inc.
295 Main Street
Mount Kisco, New York 10549

L.C. #: 83-82522
ISBN # 0-87993-207-4

This book is dedicated to my mother, Alice, and my late father, John, without whose love and sacrifice I would not have been able to achieve my life's goals.

Contributors

John G. Allison, M.D., M.B., Ch.B., FRCS(Ed), FCS(SA), FACS
Associate Professor of Surgery, Department of Surgery, Medical University of South Carolina; Chief, Surgical Services, Veterans Administration Medical Center, Charleston, South Carolina; *Formerly* Assistant Professor of Surgery, University of Iowa *and* Veterans Administration Medical Center, Iowa City, Iowa

James O. Armitage, M.D.
Associate Professor and Vice Chairman, Department of Internal Medicine, University of Nebraska Medical Center, Omaha, Nebraska

Michael P. Corder, M.D.
Associate Professor of Internal Medicine, University of Iowa, Iowa City, Iowa

Kathy Foucar, B.S., M.D.
Associate Professor, Department of Pathology, University of Iowa; Director, Electron Microscopy Laboratory, University of Iowa Hospitals and Clinics, Iowa City, Iowa

James A. Goeken, A.B., M.D.
Associate Professor, Department of Pathology, University of Iowa; Medical Director, Immunopathology Laboratory, University of Iowa Hospitals and Clinics, Iowa City, Iowa

Matthew N. Stein, M.D.
Advanced Fellow in Hematology and Oncology, Chief Resident, Department of Internal Medicine, University of Iowa Hospitals and Clinics, Iowa City, Iowa

Raymond Tannous, M.D.
Associate Professor, Hematology-Oncology Division, Department of Pediatrics, University of Iowa, Iowa City, Iowa

Hamed H. Tewfik, M.D., M.B., Ch.B., D.M.R.
Professor and Chairman, Division of Radiation Therapy, College of Medicine, University of Iowa Hospitals and Clinics, Iowa City, Iowa

Preface

The multidisciplinary treatment of cancer is a complex changing enterprise. At the present the technology is such that there is always incomplete information available; but, new information is accruing, and in particular, regarding the non-Hodgkin's lymphomas and Hodgkin's disease. In order to best deal with patients, review is necessary followed by a constant updating based on clinical research. In this manner we can deliver the most in terms of treatment, with periodic incremental satisfactory increases of success.

In the *Journal of the American Medical Association,* December 18, 1981, Dr. John G. Allison wrote a splendid essay, *The Role of Surgery in the Management of Lymphoma* in the series, "State of the Art." This multi-authored volume which follows is fabricated around many of the thoughts and principles enunciated in that essay.

The volume's thrust appears more toward the generalist than the specialist, and the verbage is conversational. With the Community Clinical Oncology Program (C-COP) coming on line, the book will be useful. Several paragraphs, in what must be construed as mainly an overall review, will be found controversial, but the reader can examine information first-hand from the references cited. And then, difference of opinion is not unhealthy.

Attention should be addressed to these important diseases and the information should be widespread to use the therapeutic advances which have been gratifying. This is in contrast to the saga of the majority of solid tumors. The histology, staging, natural history, and therapy have been addressed, even to the seemingly inconsequential (but very important) surgical biopsy. This group of essays will be useful and will find a place in our armamentarium.

ROBERT C. HICKEY, M.D. FACS
University of Texas System Cancer Center
M. D. Anderson Hospital
and Tumor Institute
Houston, Texas

Foreword

The seed of this book first stirred when my publisher, Steven Korn, read an article published in the *Journal of the American Medical Association*[1] and invited me to write a monograph on the topics encompassed by that article. The enthusiasm fired in me to do so was tempered by the realization that a publication on the role of surgery in lymphoma and gastrointestinal lymphoma only would be a slim volume indeed, with rather limited readership. It would, in addition, be incomplete, as I do not profess to be an expert in either the highly sophisticated understanding of the lymphomas' pathology or their complex current chemotherapeutic or radiotherapeutic treatment. It would be better, I thought, to invoke the special expertise of friends and colleagues and produce a complete volume that addressed all the key issues in the pathology and management of these strange malignancies of the lymphatic system. The sterling efforts by the contributing authors have fulfilled my greatest expectations and have resulted in a work that is aimed exactly where intended—not at the few score world experts in this field, but at the day-to-day working surgeon or internist, at the resident preparing for his boards, and at the medical student groping for an understanding of these confusing diseases.

The style selected is a little unusual inasmuch as there are no references cited in the text; these are to be found after each chapter as "Selected Readings." This has been done for a particular reason. Transmission of written information is enhanced by the easy flow of words and ideas, and I recall a tome I used as a medical student, one I actually enjoyed reading! I learned much while browsing through it for pleasure and hope that this book proves to be equally digestible, perhaps even as a fireside companion.

Production of a work such as this requires the diligence of many and I would like to acknowledge the efforts of all those concerned—not only those of the contributing authors, but those of all our secretaries who had to type and retype the several manuscript drafts before each chapter appeared in a form acceptable to be submitted to the publishing editors, and also the medical illustrators and photographers whose artwork grace the pages. My special thanks to Steven Korn for his invitation to edit this book and for his unflagging interest and drive to try and make us meet the deadline. I would like to acknowledge the generosity of the editors of the *Journal of the American Medical Association* for permission to reproduce, in part or in whole, passages from the article in their journal,[1] and the authors and editors for permission to reproduce a table from an article published in the *South African Medical Journal*.[2]

The successful treatment of cancer stands at Dawn's Left Hand[3] and the advances made in the treatment of the lymphomas have captured the hope and imagination of those who deal with the devastation of malignant disease. I am opposed to the practice of Medicine "by committee," but sincerely believe that the patient with cancer, lymphoma or other, can only benefit from close interdisciplinary cooperation. This volume has been compiled by physicians from several disciplines, working in just that cooperative mood. I would like to thank the authors for their contributions without which the seed would not have borne fruit. We trust that you, the reader, will enjoy reading what we have written as much as we enjoyed writing it.

JOHN G. ALLISON, M.D.

1. Allison, J.G.: The role of surgery in the management of lymphoma. *J.A.M.A.* 246:2843–2848, 1981.
2. Dent, D.M., King, H.S., and Jacobs, P.: Is staging laparotomy necessary in Hodgkin's disease? *S. African Med. J.* 65:509–511, 1982.
3. From *The Rubaiyat* of Omar Khayyam. Translated by Edward Fitzgerald.

Contents

1

Pathology of Nodal and Extranodal Lymphoma: Non-Hodgkin's Lymphoma and Hodgkin's Disease

Kathy Foucar, M.D.

Introduction

The classification and diagnosis of malignant lymphoma have undergone marked alterations in the last several decades. Although the earliest attempts at lymphoma diagnosis only emphasized distinguishing Hodgkin's disease from non-Hodgkin's lymphoma (NHL), recent advances in immunology and therapy have necessitated a more detailed classification. From its inception, there have been problems in the subclassification of malignant lymphomas, including both Hodgkin's disease and NHL. There are several reasons for these difficulties. Lymphocytes are less resistant to environmental stresses than other cell types leading to major problems with proper fixation and specimen processing. In addition, lymphocytes are dynamic cells that undergo dramatic changes in cytological features in response to antigenic stimuli, or during maturation and development. A normal lymphocyte can vary from small, with a round nucleus, to very large with a round or irregular nucleus and variably prominent nucleoli, and even progress to a plasma cell. Since lymphoreticular neoplasms mimic normal phenomena within the immune system, malignant lymphomas also exhibit a variety of cell sizes and nuclear shapes. This is especially true of NHL in which numerous cytological types have been described. Like normal lymphocytes, lymphoma cells are not stagnant and changes in the cell morphology can occur with time or can be present in different sites of disease at the same time. When one considers the triple dilemma of frequent problems with specimen preparation, the marked variety of possible cell types, and the change in cell types that frequently occurs, it becomes easier to understand the major problems that arise in the classification of malignant lymphoma, especially NHL.

Knowledge gained through immunological studies have helped the pathologist to understand the morphological diversity and heterogeneity of normal lymphocytes and related malignant lymphomas. This understanding has helped to resolve some of the dilemma in lymphoma diagnosis by making the morphological diversity more logical and predictable. Immunological studies have also increased our understanding of the natural biology of malignant lymphoma. As will be discussed in another chapter, immunological techniques allow one to identify many properties of benign and neoplastic lymphocytes and histiocytes. Such studies have elucidated the concepts of lymphocyte transformation, the term used to describe the functional and morphological changes that lymphocytes undergo in response to antigens or in maturation and development. By applying these techniques to lymphomas, it is easier to understand their morphological diversity and their types of cytological progression.

The accurate diagnosis of malignant lymphoma is obviously very important, in that major therapeutic decisions are based on the diagnosis of lymphoma not only in lymph nodes, but in a host of extranodal sites. By accurate classification of malignant lymphomas, distinct clinicopathological types have been identified. For example, certain types of NHL, including diffuse, well-differentiated lymphocytic lymphoma, have a fairly good prognosis even if no treatment is given. Other types of lymphoma, such as diffuse histiocytic lymphoma and widespread Hodgkin's disease, require aggressive multiagent chemotherapy to prevent the rapid death of the patient. Pathological staging of malignant lymphomas is as important as histological classification, in that therapy and prognosis vary with the extent (stage) of the disease. For example, the prognosis in localized (Stage I) Hodgkin's disease is clearly superior to that of disseminated (Stage IV) disease. Patients with Stage I disease may be treated with only local radiation and have an excellent survival, while patients with Stage IV disease require potent multiagent chemotherapy in order to survive. The pathologist, therefore, must be able to identify lymphoma not only in lymph node, but in bone marrow, spleen, liver, and other extranodal sites.

This chapter will discuss the morphological features of NHL and Hodgkin's disease with particular emphasis on classification. The features of involvement in lymph node, spleen, liver, and bone marrow will be illustrated. Although most cases of malignant lymphoma arise in lymph nodes, a significant fraction arises in extranodal sites such as the gastrointestinal (GI) tract, lung, skin, and head and neck regions. The lymphomas that arise in these areas will be discussed as well as features that help to distinguish lymphoma from "pseudolymphoma" in extranodal sites.

Non-Hodgkin's Lymphoma

Classification of NHL

Non-Hodgkin's lymphomas arise from the autonomous proliferation of B lymphocytes, T lymphocytes, lymphocytes without identifiable immunological features ("null" lymphocytes), and occasionally from true histiocytes (macrophages). In addition to these immunological cell types, the neoplastic lymphocytes can assume various sizes and shapes corresponding to the stages of transformation and maturation as discussed above. Earlier classification schemes for the NHLs were based on the cytological features of the tumor cells, as well as the pattern of nodal infiltration which was described as either nodular or diffuse. One such classification system, proposed by Rappaport in the 1950s and later modified, has since become the most widely used for NHL in the United States. Although some of the terminology in the Rappaport classification has been shown to be incorrect by immunological techniques, its widespread use and clinical relevance make it the system of choice for this chapter. More recent and immunologically precise classification systems will be briefly reviewed and compared with the Rappaport system. Some of the newer terms will be incorporated in this morphological description of the Rappaport system in an attempt to update this classification and facilitate correlation with the newer classifications, most notably the Working Formulation for clinical usage.

Rappaport Classification of NHL (Table 1)

Well-differentiated Lymphocytic Lymphoma (WDLL) *[Malignant lymphoma, small lymphocytic in Working Formulation]*

The modified Rappaport classification of NHL is shown on Table 1. In this classification, the lymphoid-appearing cells are classified as

Table 1
Modified Rappaport Classification of Non-Hodgkin's Lymphoma

Cell Types	*Growth Pattern**
Well-differentiated lymphocytic lymphoma	Diffuse
Intermediately differentiated lymphocytic lymphoma	Diffuse, Nodular
Poorly differentiated lymphocytic lymphoma	Nodular, Diffuse
Mixed lymphocytic-histiocytic lymphoma	Diffuse, Nodular
Histiocytic lymphoma	Diffuse, Nodular
Undifferentiated, Burkitt's and non-Burkitt's	Diffuse, Nodular†
Lymphoblastic	Diffuse

*Most common pattern given first
†Nodular pattern is extremely rare

well, intermediately, or poorly differentiated, and the pattern of nodal infiltration is designated as nodular or diffuse. WDLL is a malignant lymphoma comprised of a fairly monotonous population of small, lymphocytes with round nuclear contours, dense chromatin, inconspicuous nucleoli, and scant cytoplasm (Figs. 1, 2). Occasionally larger cells with variably prominent nucleoli and a moderate amount of cytoplasm are seen. These large cells, called prolymphocytes and blast-like cells, can be evenly dispersed among the more numerous small

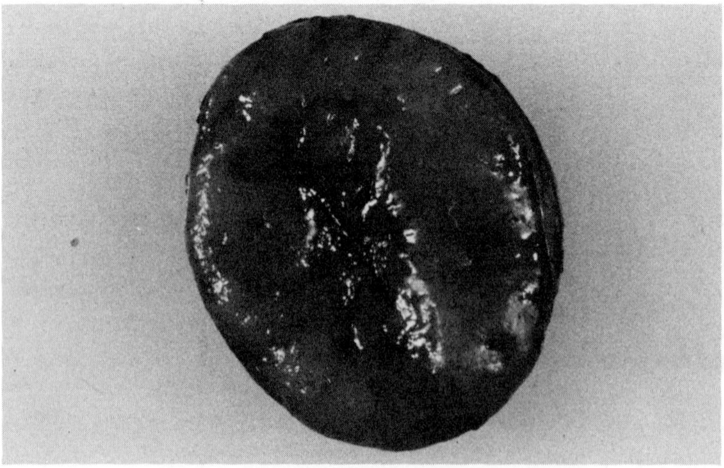

Figure 1: This gross photograph of a lymph node shows the typical homogeneous, fish-flesh pattern of malignant lymphoma. No areas of necrosis are identified.

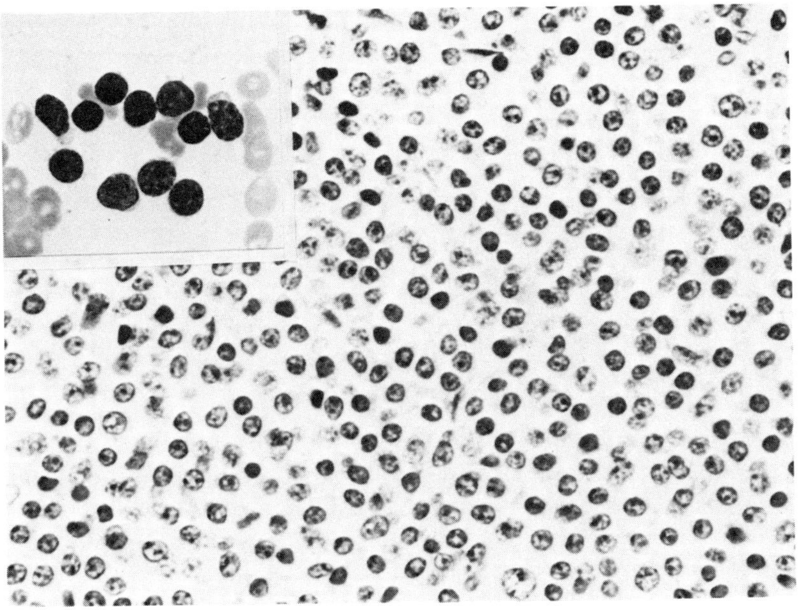

Figure 2: This high power view of WDLL involving a lymph node shows a monotonous infiltrate of small round lymphocytes with only occasional larger prolymphocytes and blast-like cells. *Inset:* WDLL in bone marrow in which a monotonous population of mature appearing lymphocytes is noted.

lymphocytes or form aggregates called pseudofollicular growth centers. These larger cells represent the proliferative component of the lymphoma; the small lymphocytes lack mitotic capability. The pattern of nodal infiltration in WDLL is almost always diffuse. As shown on Table 2, this type of NHL is relatively uncommon. Most commonly affected are middle-aged to elderly males.

Splenic, hepatic, and bone marrow infiltration are fairly frequent in WDLL. The earliest infiltrates within the spleen are localized to the white pulp follicles, but eventual red pulp infiltration occurs. Hepatic infiltrates are first identified in the portal tracts. The reported frequency of bone marrow involvement at the time of diagnosis varies greatly but is generally high. Bone marrow infiltrates tend to form small, randomly placed foci within the medullary cavity, and the extent of bone marrow replacement by the lymphoma is usually not great. In all of these extranodal disease sites, the lymphoma cells have essentially the same cytological features as those described in the lymph node (Fig. 2). Cytologically and histologically, bone marrow and

Table 2
Frequency of NHL According to Rappaport Classification

Morphological Type	*% NHL*
WDLL, diffuse	4
PDLL, nodular	17
PDLL, diffuse	11
Mixed lymphocytic-histiocytic, nodular	18
Mixed lymphocytic-histiocytic, diffuse	10
Histiocytic, nodular	7
Histiocytic, diffuse	30
Undifferentiated, diffuse	3

blood involvement by WDLL can be virtually identical to chronic lymphocytic leukemia (CLL). The distinction between WDLL and CLL is based on the presence of a prominent (>5,000) peripheral blood lymphocytosis in CLL. Occasionally patients with WDLL develop aggressive lymphoma comprised of large cells that are immunologically similar to the WDLL.

Intermediately Differentiated Lymphocytic Lymphoma (IDLL)

IDLL is a fairly recently proposed type of NHL that affects predominantly adults. This type of lymphoma is not included in all studies using the Rappaport classification. In IDLL, the lymphoma cells are somewhat larger than those of WDLL, and they exhibit some nuclear irregularity although it is not pronounced. Indeed, these cells have cytological features intermediate between the small round lymphocytes of WDLL and the small cleaved cells of poorly differentiated lymphocytic lymphoma (PDLL). The lymphoma cell nuclei have dense chromatin, variable nucleoli, and scant to moderate amounts of cytoplasm (Fig. 3). Mitotic activity is variable and may be prominent. The pattern of nodal infiltration is usually diffuse, although a nodular variant has been described. The nodular variant is thought to arise from the mantle zone of lymphocytes which surrounds germinal centers in a lymph node.

Splenic involvement is initially localized to the white pulp follicles, and hepatic involvement is localized in the portal tracts. There is a high frequency of bone marrow and blood involvement in IDLL; occasionally patients present with a leukemic blood profile with a markedly elevated white count, anemia, and/or thrombocytopenia. These circulating lymphoma cells have nuclei ranging from round to

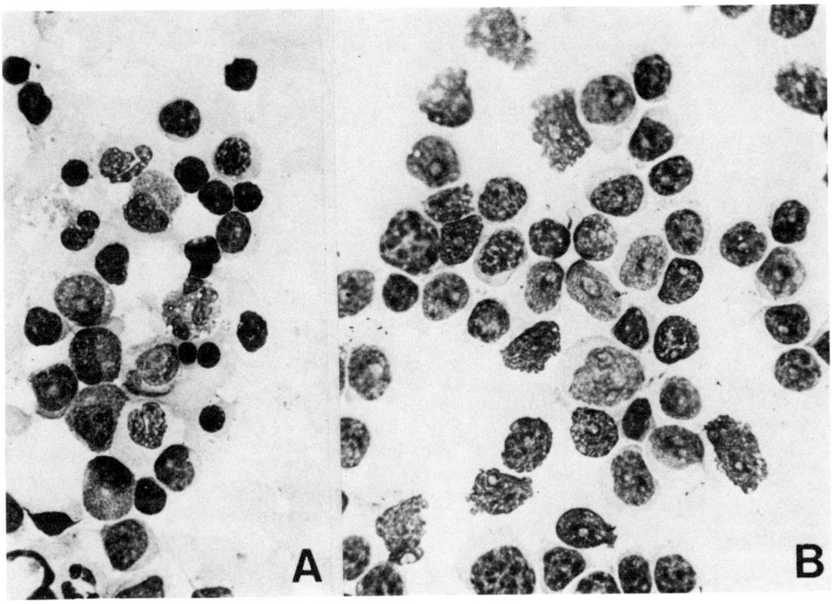

Figure 3: The cytologic features of IDLL cells in bone marrow aspirate (A) and lymph node imprint smear (B) are shown. These lymphoma cells vary in size and some nuclear irregularity is evident. In this particular case, nucleoli are fairly prominent.

irregular with a fair proportion of cleaved forms. The amount of cytoplasm is usually moderate (Fig. 3). The extent of bone marrow replacement is variable, but can be quite high, and the lymphomatous infiltrate can be randomly located within the medullary cavity or molded against bony trabeculae (paratrabecular).

Poorly Differentiated Lymphocytic Lymphoma (PDLL) [Malignant lymphoma, follicular and/or diffuse, small cleaved cell in Working Formulation]

PDLL is a common type of NHL (Table 2) that affects adults and shows a male predominance. In PDLL, the lymphoma cells are larger than those of WDLL and have nuclei that are distinctly irregular and cleaved. These cells have recently been named "small cleaved cells" because their nuclei are smaller than macrophage nuclei and nuclear irregularity is pronounced. Lymphoma cells of this type are similar to cells of non-neoplastic germinal centers where marked nuclear irregularity is a consistent cytological feature. The nuclear clefts of

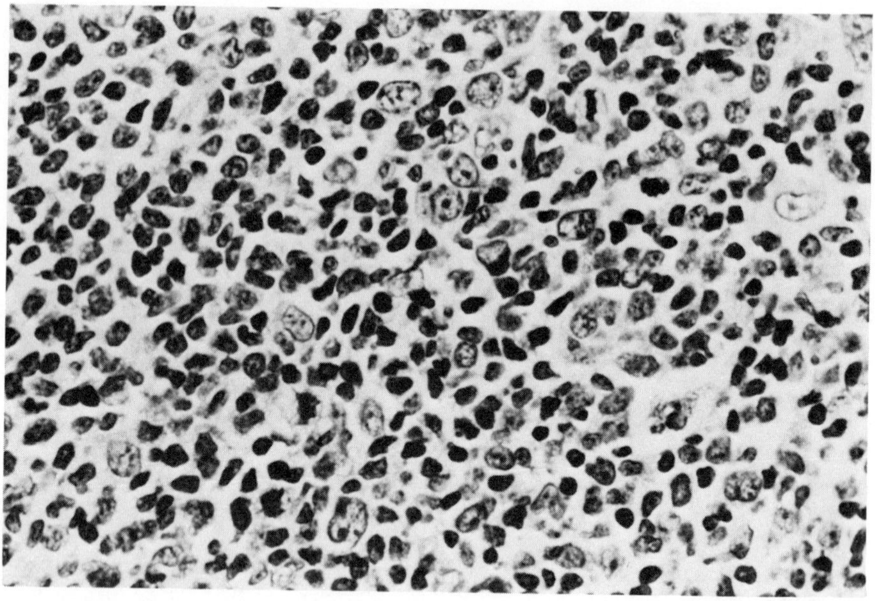

Figure 4: This high power view of a lymph node with nodular PDLL shows a marked predominance of small cleaved cells. These cells exhibit prominent nuclear irregularity, have dense nuclear chromatin, and inconspicuous cytoplasm. In addition, small numbers of large cells are identified. These cells generally have round nuclei and one to two nuclei (large noncleaved cells). Occasional large cleaved cells are noted also.

PDLL frequently divide the nucleus almost into two separate lobes. The nuclear chromatin of these cells is dense and nucleoli are inconspicuous. The cells have minimal to moderate amounts of cytoplasm (Figs. 4, 8). Other newly named large cell types which are consistently identified in PDLL ("large cleaved" and "large noncleaved" cells) are also analogous to the cells seen in non-neoplastic germinal centers (Fig. 4). Mitotic activity is generally minimal in PDLL and is roughly proportional to the number of large cells present. The pattern of nodal infiltration is commonly nodular (follicular), again attesting to the relationship of PDLL to germinal center cells (Fig. 5). A fair number of these nodular lymphomas will become diffuse during the later disease course. Occasionally a diffuse pattern of infiltration is seen at presentation in PDLL.

Splenic, hepatic, and bone marrow involvement are frequent at presentation in PDLL. The spleen shows initial involvement of the white pulp follicles (Figs. 6, 7), the liver shows predominantly portal tract infiltration, and the bone marrow shows a variable extent of

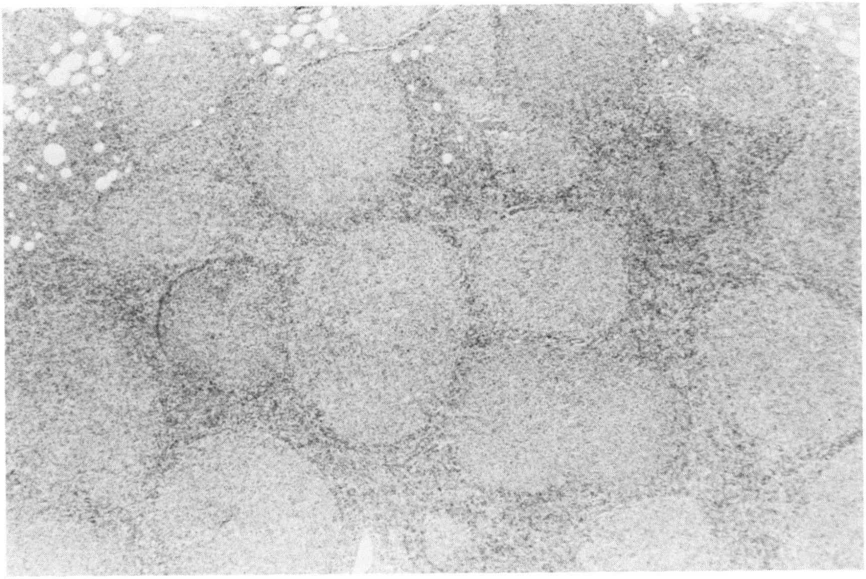

Figure 5: This low power photomicrograph of nodular PDLL shows the closely spaced nodules typical of this type of lymphoma. Note that the nodules extend into the perinodal adipose tissue.

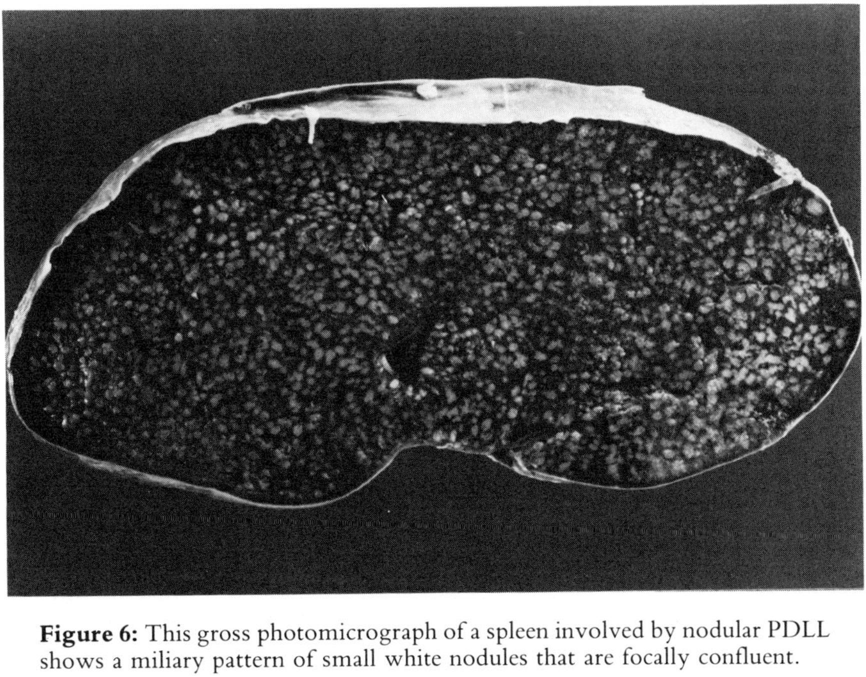

Figure 6: This gross photomicrograph of a spleen involved by nodular PDLL shows a miliary pattern of small white nodules that are focally confluent.

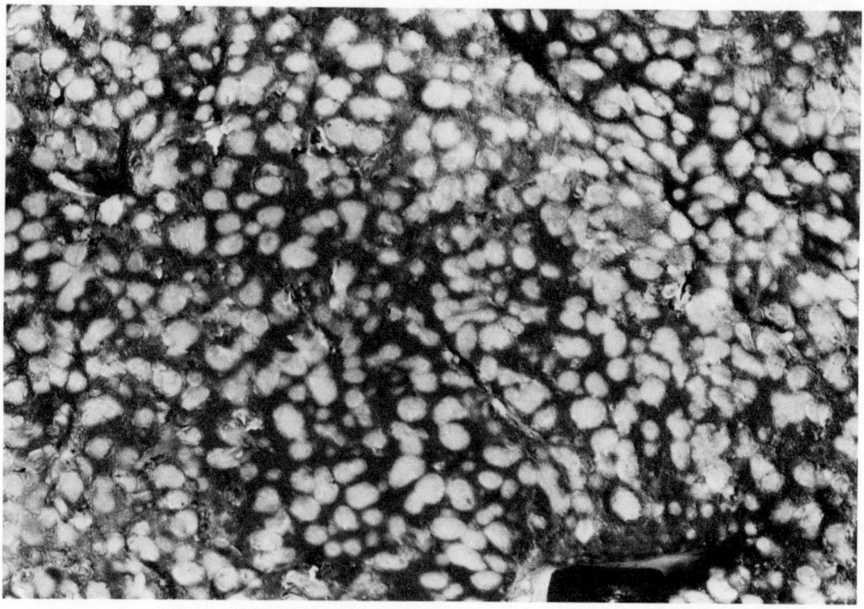

Figure 7: This closeup view of the same spleen as in Figure 6 shows the numerous distinct white nodular infiltrates of lymphoma, most of which are approximately the same size.

replacement by lymphoma cells showing a distinct propensity to mold against bony trabeculae (Fig. 8). This paratrabecular bone marrow pattern of infiltration is characteristic of nodular PDLL. In all these sites the predominant cell is typically the small cleaved cell, identical to that seen in the lymph node (Fig. 8). Occasionally large cleaved or large noncleaved cells predominate in these extranodal sites, even though the nodal disease contained mostly small cleaved cells. Likewise, the small cleaved cell population may eventually be replaced by large cells in all sites. These phenomena are compatible with the concept of lymphocyte transformation in which the morphology of the lymphoma can differ in various sites of disease or change with time.

Mixed Lymphocytic–Histiocytic Lymphoma [Malignant lymphoma, follicular and/or diffuse, mixed small and large cell in Working Formulation]

Rappaport used the phrase "mixed lymphocytic-histiocytic" to describe a lymphoma comprised of both small and large cells, neither

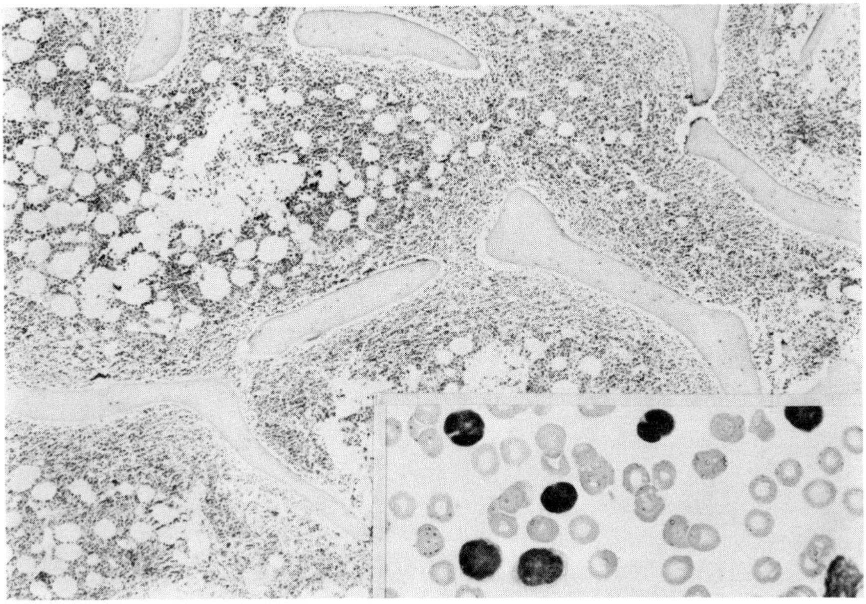

Figure 8: This medium power photomicrograph of bone marrow involved by nodular PDLL shows a prominent paratrabecular pattern to the lymphomatous infiltrate. *Inset:* circulating lymphoma cells from the same patient. Note the marked nuclear clefting, dense nuclear chromatin, and scant cytoplasm.

of which predominate. Mixed lymphomas are fairly common (Table 2), affecting predominantly adults. The small lymphocyte nuclei are usually irregular and in some cases are cleaved. The large cell component, designated as "histiocytic" in the Rappaport system, is one of transformed lymphocytes. In mixed lymphoma with a nodular pattern of infiltration, the small cells have cleaved nuclei identical to the small cleaved cells in PDLL cells and the large cells are large cleaved and/or large noncleaved cells, which, although more numerous, are similar to those seen in nodular PDLL (Figs. 9, 10).

Those cases of diffuse mixed lymphocytic-histiocytic lymphoma are a more heterogeneous and complex group. Although some are the diffuse counterpart of nodular mixed lymphomas, other types of lymphoma are included within this category. For example, WDLL, in which there are large numbers of transformed cells, would result in a mixed lymphoma because of the admixture of small and large cells. In addition, a variety of lymphomas derived from mature, post-thymic (sometimes called peripheral) T lymphocytes are characteris-

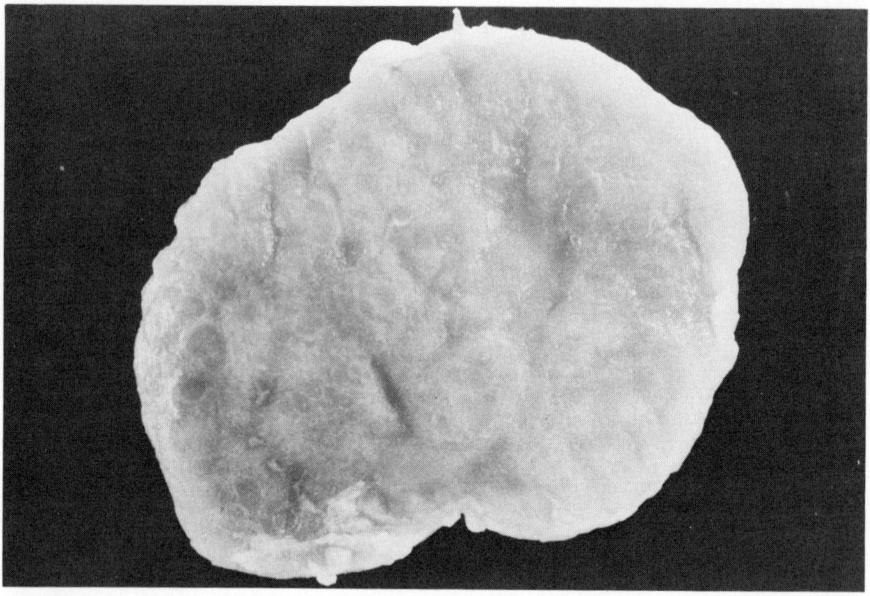

Figure 9: Multiple small nodules are apparent in this gross photograph of a nodular mixed lymphocytic-histiocytic lymphoma.

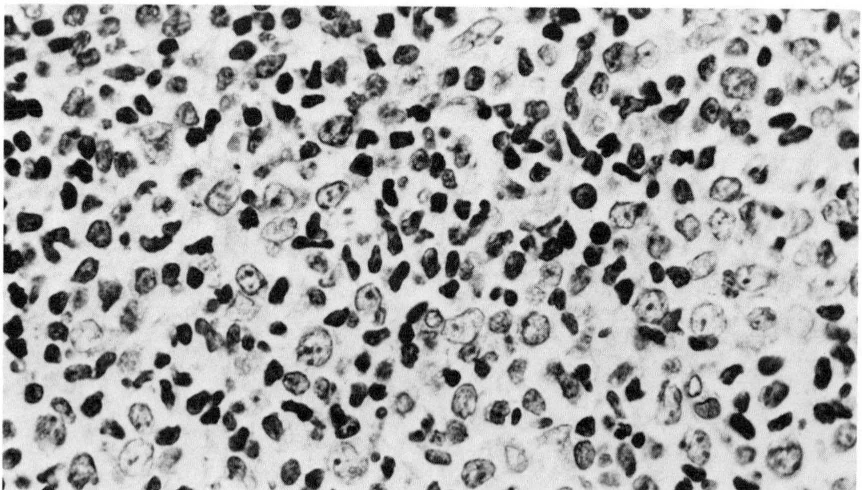

Figure 10: This high power photomicrograph of nodular mixed lymphocytic-histiocytic lymphoma shows a mixed population of small cleaved cells and larger cleaved and noncleaved cells. The large cell population is clearly more generous than noted in nodular PDLL.

tically comprised of both small and large cells (Fig. 11). Other cell types such as eosinophils, plasma cells, and epithelioid true histiocytes are commonly present in peripheral T-cell lymphomas, further adding to the mixed nature of the process. Included among peripheral T-cell lymphomas are such distinct clinicopathologic entities as Lennert's (lymphoepithelioid cell) lymphoma and a group of mixed lymphomas described by Waldron et al.

There is variable involvement of spleen, liver, and bone marrow in mixed lymphomas. Although there are few reports describing the involvement of these organs in nodular mixed lymphocytic-histiocytic lymphoma, they can be expected to parallel those described for nodular PDLL, except for the larger component of large cleaved and large noncleaved cells. Bone marrow involvement, however, is not as common in nodular mixed lymphocytic-histiocytic lymphoma as it is in nodular PDLL. The features of diffuse mixed lymphoma in spleen, liver, and bone marrow are not well described. Bone marrow infiltrates, when present, consist of focal infiltrates randomly scattered

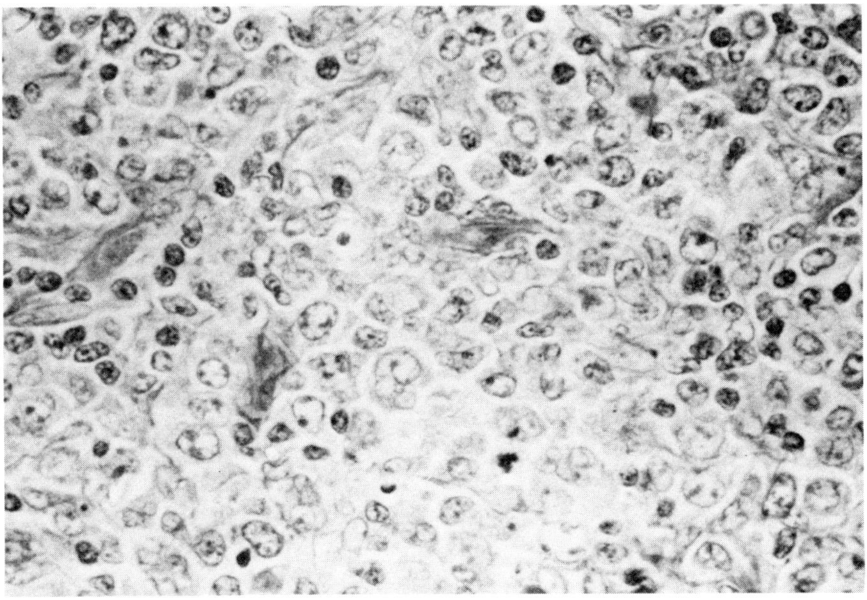

Figure 11: This high power photomicrograph of a peripheral T-cell lymphoma shows a polymorphous infiltrate of small and large cells. The large cells have vesicular nuclei and prominent lobulation is identified in some. Vascular proliferation is also evident.

throughout the medullary cavity or diffuse, extensive infiltrates with large areas of architectural obliteration.

Histiocytic Lymphoma [Malignant lymphoma, follicular and/or diffuse, large cell (cleaved or noncleaved) or large cell, immunoblastic in Working Formulation]

Histiocytic lymphomas, especially those with a diffuse pattern of infiltration, are a very common type of NHL (Table 2). Rappaport used the term "histiocytic" to describe those lymphomas comprised of cells with nuclei the same size as or larger than macrophage nuclei. Recent immunological characterization shows that the vast majority of these lymphomas are actually derived from transformed lymphocytes. Only a rare case of histiocytic lymphoma is comprised of histiocytes. More recent terminology, which will be discussed later, has

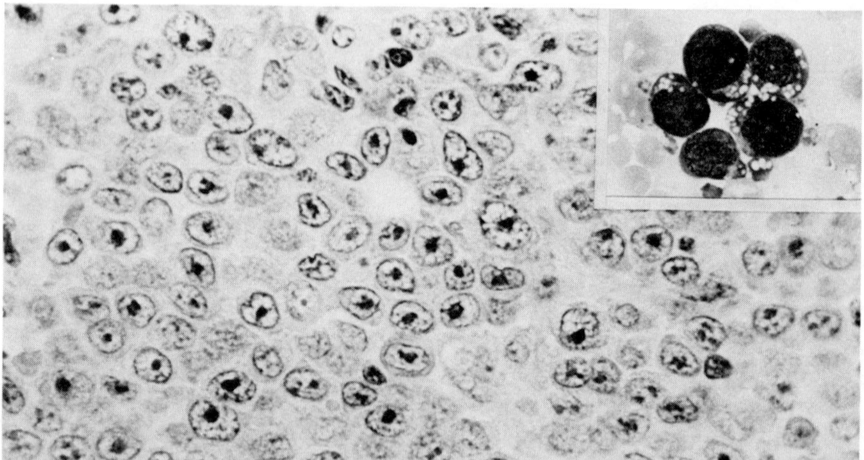

Figure 12: This high power photomicrograph of a lymph node involved by diffuse histiocytic lymphoma shows a marked predominance of large noncleaved cells. These cells have generally round nuclear contours, prominent nucleoli, and vesicular nuclear chromatin. Cytoplasm is evident but not prominent. *Inset:* bone marrow aspirate from same patient shows involvement by lymphoma. The lymphoma cell nuclei are round, nucleoli are apparent, and the moderate cytoplasm contains numerous vacuoles.

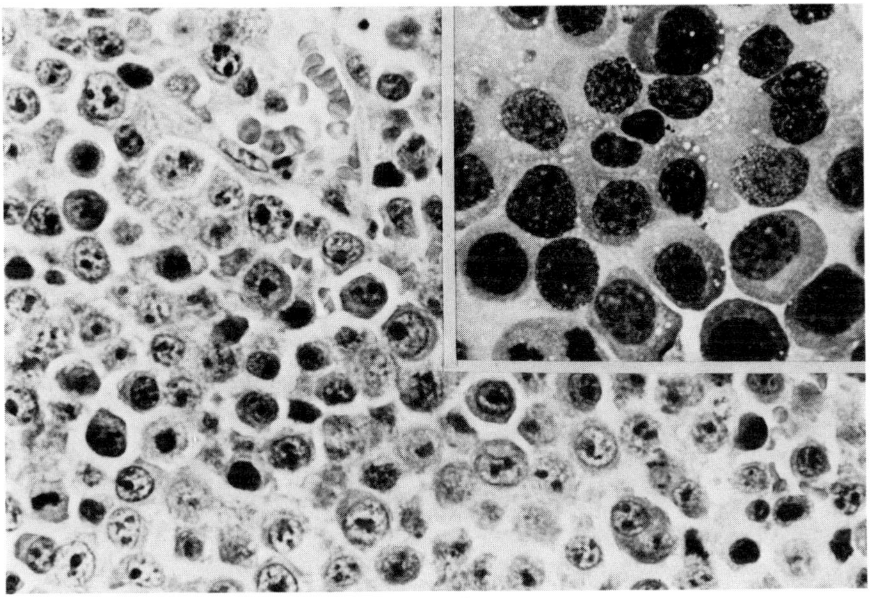

Figure 13: This high power photomicrograph of a lymph node with diffuse histiocytic lymphoma is comprised of large cells with morphologic features of immunoblasts. The nuclei vary somewhat in size, are round, the nucleoli are quite conspicuous, and the cytoplasm is abundant and pyroninophilic. *Inset:* touch preparations from this lymph node show obvious plasmacellular differentiation. The amount of cytoplasm is abundant, the nuclei are somewhat eccentric, and a spectrum between smaller plasma cells and the large immunoblasts is evident.

separated Rappaport's histiocytic lymphomas into large cleaved cell, large noncleaved cell, and immunoblastic cell subtypes. As the names imply, the large cleaved cells have distinct nuclear clefts similar to the small cleaved cells while the large noncleaved cells have round nuclear contours. Nucleoli can be seen in both of these cell types, but are more prominent in large noncleaved cells. The amount of cytoplasm is moderate in the large noncleaved cells and is usually less obvious in the large cleaved cells. The large cleaved and large noncleaved cells are identical to those described in PDLL, but they predominate, with the small cleaved (PDLL) cell being inconspicuous or absent (Figs. 4, 10, 12) The large immunoblastic cell tends to have a large round to lobated nucleus with fairly prominent, centrally located nucleoli, and a moderate amount of basophilic cytoplasm. In some immunoblastic lymphomas, cells with features of plasma cells and features intermediate between plasma cells and immunoblasts are seen (Fig. 13). Large

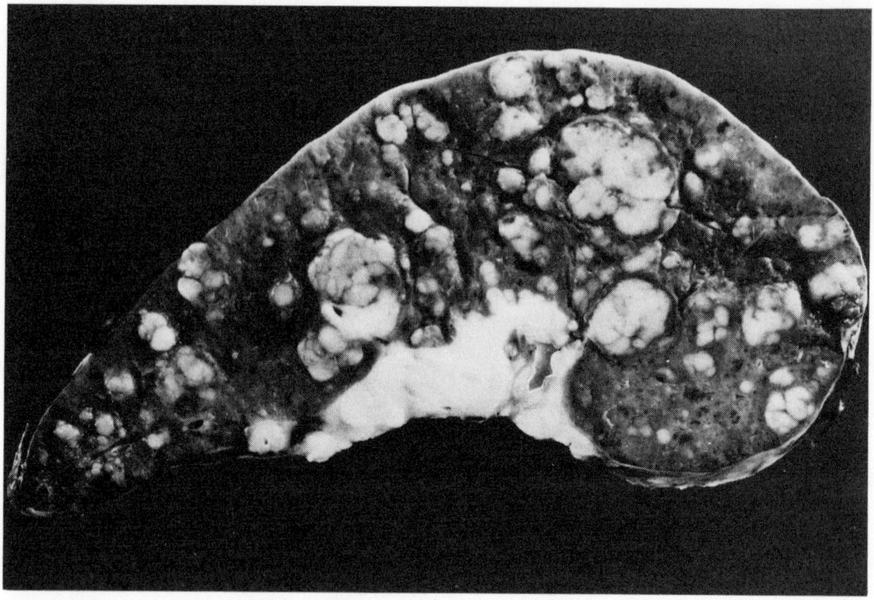

Figure 14: This gross photograph of a spleen shows extensive involvement by diffuse histiocytic lymphoma manifested by multiple large mass lesions. There is also extensive involvement of the hilar lymph nodes adjacent to the spleen.

cell lymphomas of any of the types described above are frequently diffuse, although occasional cases of large cleaved or large noncleaved cell lymphoma have a nodular growth pattern, attesting to their relationship to non-neoplastic germinal center cells.

Histiocytic lymphoma in spleen, liver, and bone marrow at presentation is relatively uncommon. When present in the spleen, histiocytic lymphomas tend to form large mass lesions, with extensive areas of architectural destruction (Fig. 14). Those occasional cases in which the bone marrow is involved at presentation show small focal aggregates of lymphoma cells. Diffuse infiltration of bone marrow elements occurs rarely. These lymphomatous infiltrates are usually cytologically similar to those seen in the lymph nodes, although some exceptions do occur (Fig. 12).

Undifferentiated, Burkitt's and Non-Burkitt's [Malignant lymphoma, diffuse, small noncleaved cell in Working Formulation]

Undifferentiated lymphomas (an infrequent type of NHL) are comprised of mitotically active cells that range from intermediate to large in size. Depending upon the uniformity of the lymphomatous infiltrate, the tumors are designated as Burkitt's (when cells are quite uniform) or non-Burkitt's (when cells are heterogeneous). A more recent term for undifferentiated lymphoma is "small noncleaved cell lymphoma." Undifferentiated lymphoma, Burkitt's type, represents a clinicopathological entity first described in African children which shows a propensity for extranodal involvement . Lymphomas with histological features identical to African Burkitt's lymphoma have been described in the United States and in various other countries. American Burkitt's lymphoma occurs in a slightly older child than the African type and also shows frequent extranodal involvement (Fig. 15). In all sites of involvement by Burkitt's lymphoma the cells have uniformly round nuclei with stippled chromatin and multiple small, but distinct, nucleoli. There is a moderate amount of deeply basophilic cytoplasm containing numerous sharply demarcated lipid vacuoles (Fig. 15). Prominent mitotic activity is common with numerous be-

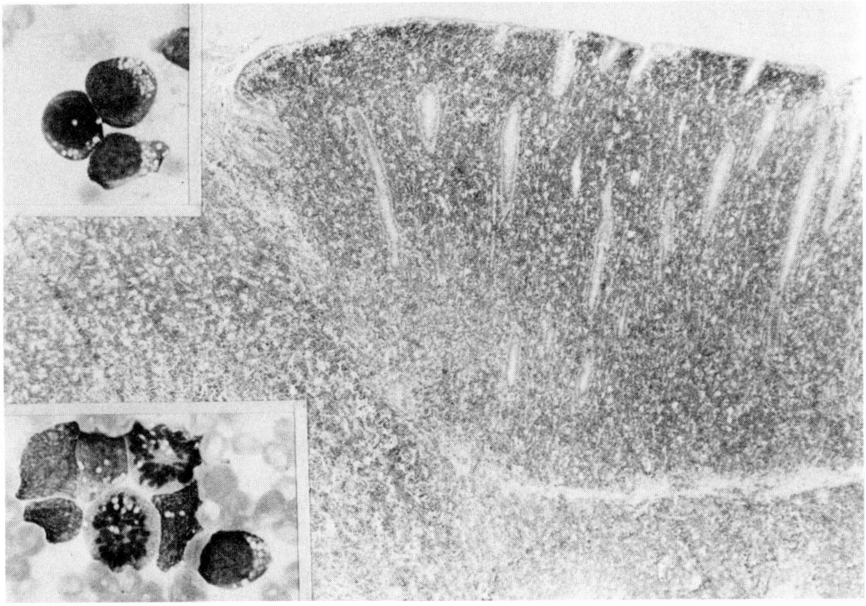

Figure 15: This medium power photomicrograph of ileum shows an extensive infiltrate by Burkitt's lymphoma. A few residual glands are evident. The "starry sky" pattern noted is due to the large numbers of macrophages within the tumor. *Insets:* the cytologic details of these tumor cells are shown. The nuclei are medium-sized and round. The cytoplasm is moderate in amount, deeply basophilic, and contains distinct cytoplasmic vacuoles. Several mitoses are evident on these imprint preparations.

nign macrophages intermixed with the lymphoma, imparting a "starry sky" appearance. The pattern of nodal infiltration is virtually always diffuse, although a very rare case with a focally nodular pattern has been described.

Undifferentiated, non-Burkitt's lymphomas are similar to Burkitt's lymphoma except for greater variation in nuclear size and shape, with fewer, more prominent nucleoli. Undifferentiated, non-Burkitt's lymphomas tend to occur in a wider age range and many patients are adults. Undifferentiated, non-Burkitt's lymphomas likewise have a propensity for extranodal presentation; especially common is GI tract disease. The clinical and cytological features are similar enough to suggest that these two undifferentiated (small noncleaved cell) lymphomas are variants of the same disease. However, the marked association of Epstein-Barr virus infection with African Burkitt's lymphoma is less frequent in Burkitt's and undifferentiated non-Burkitt's lymphomas from other geographic areas.

The liver and spleen are uncommon sites of involvement in either type of undifferentiated (small noncleaved cell) lymphoma at the time of presentation. Autopsy findings of extensive multiple organ system disease are common. Bone marrow involvement may occur late in the course of disease and is usually one of extensive replacement by cells similar to those described in other sites (Fig. 15). Despite extensive bone marrow replacement, leukemic blood findings are uncommon. A rare case of acute lymphoblastic leukemia with cells indistinguishable from Burkitt's lymphoma cells has, however, been described.

Lymphoblastic Lymphoma [Malignant lymphoma, lymphoblastic in Working Formulation]

Lymphoblastic lymphoma, originally classified as diffuse PDLL, is comprised of variably sized cells that commonly exhibit nuclear irregularity and have finely stippled, dusty, nuclear chromatin with inconspicuous nucleoli. The cytoplasm is scant and may contain glycogen and the enzyme, acid phosphatase (Fig. 16). Mitotic activity is brisk, and increased numbers of benign macrophages may impart a "starry sky" appearance. The pattern of lymph node involvement is always diffuse. Like Burkitt's lymphoma, lymphoblastic lymphoma appears to represent a distinct clinicopathological entity which is associated with marked male predominance, frequent occurrence in teenagers and young adults, and mediastinal mass formation. Lymphoblastic lymphoma has been described in older patients in whom it

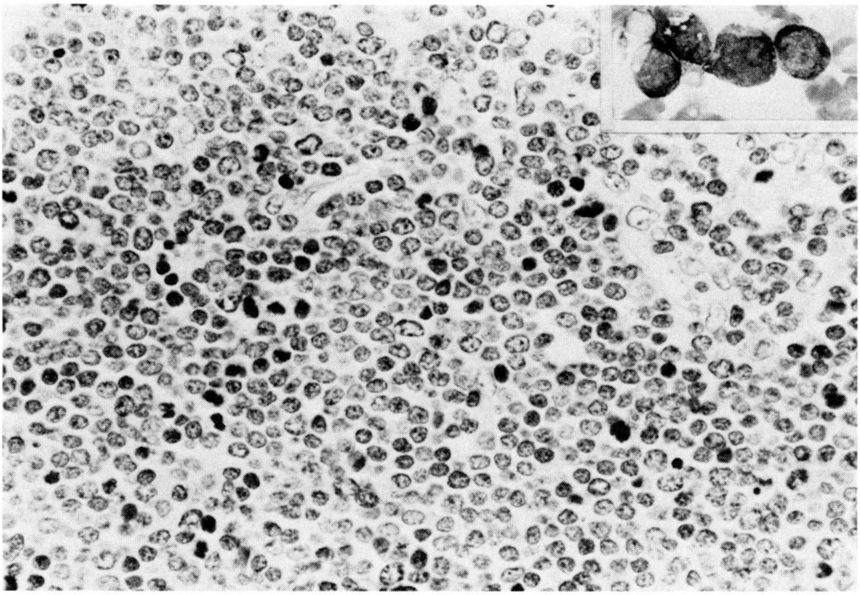

Figure 16: This high power photomicrograph of a lymph node involved by lymphoblastic lymphoma shows cells with finely stippled nuclear chromatin, indistinct nucleoli, and scant cytoplasm. Mitotic activity is brisk. *Inset:* the bone marrow from this patient shows an infiltrate of variably sized lymphoblast-like cells with moderate to scant cytoplasm. Nuclear irregularity is evident.

does not show the marked predilection for mediastinal mass formation. Widespread lymph node disease with progression to blood and bone marrow involvement is common, especially in the younger age group.

There appears to be a significant clinical and morphological overlap between lymphoblastic lymphoma and a subgroup of acute lymphoblastic leukemia (ALL) which is comprised of T (or sometimes null cell) lymphoblasts. On lymph node imprint preparations and bone marrow smears, the cells of lymphoblastic lymphoma are indistinguishable from the blast cells of ALL (Fig. 16). Bone marrow involvement in lymphoblastic lymphoma can be extensive and show a diffuse interstitial ("leukemic") pattern, identical to ALL. The distinction between lymphoblastic lymphoma and ALL is usually made on clinical grounds. Those cases with dominant lymph node disease are called lymphoblastic lymphoma, while those with major bone marrow and blood involvement associated with significant anemia and/or thrombocytopenia are called ALL. Splenomegaly is more frequent in ALL. The distinction is occasionally impossible to make. Recent immunological data suggest a subtle difference between lymphoblastic lymphoma and T-ALL, but the sophisticated methods needed to make this distinction are not widely available.

Other Classification Systems

During the 1970s, multiple classification systems for NHL were proposed. Reasons for this plethora of classifications related, in part, to immunological studies of NHL which offered a new dimension in lymphoma diagnosis and which demonstrated some imprecisions in the Rappaport classification system. Systems were proposed by the World Health Organization, Drs. Dorfman, Lennert, Bennett-Farrar and Henry, and Lukes and Collins. Some of these systems attempted to correlate morphology with immunology and some promoted the morphological concepts of lymphocyte transformation discussed earlier. None gained widespread use in the United States, except possibly the classification by Lukes and Collins. Because of the multiple competing classification systems, compounded by the already existing difficulties in the consistent diagnosis of NHL, there developed significant problems in comparing data on NHL from different institutions. Partly because of these problems, a large study was conducted in which numerous cases of NHL were blindly reviewed by panels of hematopathologists and experienced surgical pathologists. All of the proposed classification systems were applied to each case. All of the classifications were shown to have clinical relevance, but none was found to be superior to the others. A Working Formulation for Clinical Usage was proposed to facilitate comparisons between institutions, and to provide a universal classification system with which all others could be compared and interchanged.

Working Formulation for Clinical Usage (Table 3)

The Working Formulation is an attempt by hematopathologists and clinicians to incorporate the most favorable features of earlier classification systems, including those that have proven clinical significance. The terminology used in the classification correlates well

Table 3
Working Formulation for Clinical Usage and Incidence of NHL†

Low grade	*% of NHL*
Malignant lymphoma (ML), small lymphocytic	4
ML, follicular, predominantly small cleaved cell	22
ML, follicular, mixed small cleaved and large cell	8
Intermediate grade	
ML, follicular, predominantly large cell	4
ML, diffuse, small cleaved cell	7
ML, diffuse, mixed small and large cell	7
ML, diffuse, large cell	20
• cleaved cell	
• noncleaved cell	
High grade	
ML, large cell, immunoblastic	8
• plasmacytoid	
• clear cell	
• polymorphous	
• epithelioid cell component	
ML, lymphoblastic	4
ML, small noncleaved cell	5
• Burkitt's	
Miscellaneous	11
Composite lymphoma	
Mycosis fungoides	
Histiocytic	
Extramedullary plasmacytoma	
Unclassifiable	
Other	

†From: The non-Hodgkin's lymphoma pathologic classification project: National Cancer Institute sponsored study of classifications of non-Hodgkin's lymphomas–Summary and description of a working formulation for clinical usage. *Cancer* 49:2112–2135, 1982.

with current immunological information. The Working Formulation includes both clinical and pathological features of NHL. The lymphoma subtypes are divided into low, intermediate, and high grade groups based on the clinical course of each (Table 3). Within each grade are several morphological subtypes, classified according to cell type and pattern of nodal infiltration. The Working Formulation uses some cytological terms designed to define lymphocyte transformation within the germinal center, and omits terms (such as "histiocytic") that are immunologically incorrect. The cell types include small lymphocytic, small cleaved cell, large cell (large cleaved, large noncleaved, and immunoblastic), lymphoblastic, and small noncleaved cell. The details of these cytological types have been described in the section on the Rappaport classification.

The pattern of nodal infiltration (either follicular or diffuse) is an integral part of the Working Formulation because of evidence confirming better survival for patients with follicular lymphoma when compared with patients with diffuse lymphoma of the same cell type. "Follicular" is synonymous with "nodular" in the Rappaport system, and was chosen to emphasize the relationship between follicular lymphomas and normal lymph node follicles (germinal centers). This has been confirmed by immunological, cytochemical, and ultrastructural studies.

Table 4 compares the Working Formulation with the Rappaport classification system. Familiarity with this comparison is important since an adoption of the Working Formulation by pathologists throughout the country would force physicians to understand and interconvert between systems. Although this book utilizes the Rappaport system, I have deliberately used terminology proposed by the Working Formulation in the description of each Rappaport subtype in an attempt to facilitate interconversion between the two systems.

Table 4
Comparison of Rappaport Classification and Working Formulation for Major Types of NHL†

Rappaport Classification★		*Working Formulation*
WDLL	→	Malignant lymphoma (ML), small lymphocytic
IDLL	→ (to small lymphocytic and to diffuse, small cleaved cell)	
PDLL, nodular	→	ML, follicular, small cleaved cell
Mixed, lymphocytic-histiocytic nodular	→	ML, follicular, mixed small cleaved and large cell
Histiocytic, nodular	→	ML, follicular, large cell
PDLL, diffuse	→	ML, diffuse, small cleaved cell
Mixed lymphocytic-histiocytic diffuse	→	ML, diffuse, mixed small and large cell
DHL	→	ML, diffuse, large cell
	→	ML, large cell, immunoblastic
	→	ML, histiocytic
Lymphoblastic	→	ML, lymphoblastic
Undifferentiated, Burkitt's and non-Burkitt's	→	ML, small noncleaved cell

†Abbreviations in text
★Arrow = morphologically corresponds to

Relative Frequencies of NHL in Adults and Children

NHL is much more common in adults than in children. The most frequent types of NHL encountered in adults are nodular PDLL (follicular small cleaved cell lymphoma), nodular mixed lymphocytic-histiocytic lymphoma (follicular, mixed small cleaved, and large cell) and diffuse large cell lymphomas. In contrast, nodular (follicular) lymphomas and WDLL are extremely uncommon in children. The most frequent types reported in children include lymphoblastic lymphoma, undifferentiated (small noncleaved cell) lymphoma, and diffuse large cell lymphoma.

Hodgkin's Disease

Reed-Sternberg Cells

Hodgkin's disease is the uncontrolled proliferation of a distinctive large cell and its variants. Following detailed morphological descriptions of this cell around the turn of the century by Sternberg and Reed, this cell has since been called the Reed-Sternberg (RS) cell. The typical RS cell is a very large multinucleated or multilobated cell with huge central, eosinophilic nucleoli. There is perinucleolar clearing of the nuclear chromatin, and the cytoplasm of the RS cell is generally abundant (Fig. 17). A variety of mononuclear and multinucleated RS variants have also been described. Cytogenetic studies demonstrate aneuploidy (an excess of DNA) of RS cells and RS variants documenting their neoplastic nature. The origin of the RS cells is controversial and evidence has been published to support multiple cells of origin. These include B cells, T cells, monocyte-macrophages, interdigitating reticulum cells, and even an (as yet) undefined cell. This controversy will be discussed in more detail in the chapter on immunology (Chapter 2) in which the evidence to support or refute the various cells of origin proposed for Hodgkin's disease will be presented.

General Features of Hodgkin's Disease

Hodgkin's disease arises almost exclusively in lymph nodes, predominantly in the neck; a pure extranodal presentation of Hodgkin's disease is distinctly rare. Many detailed studies of staging in Hodgkin's

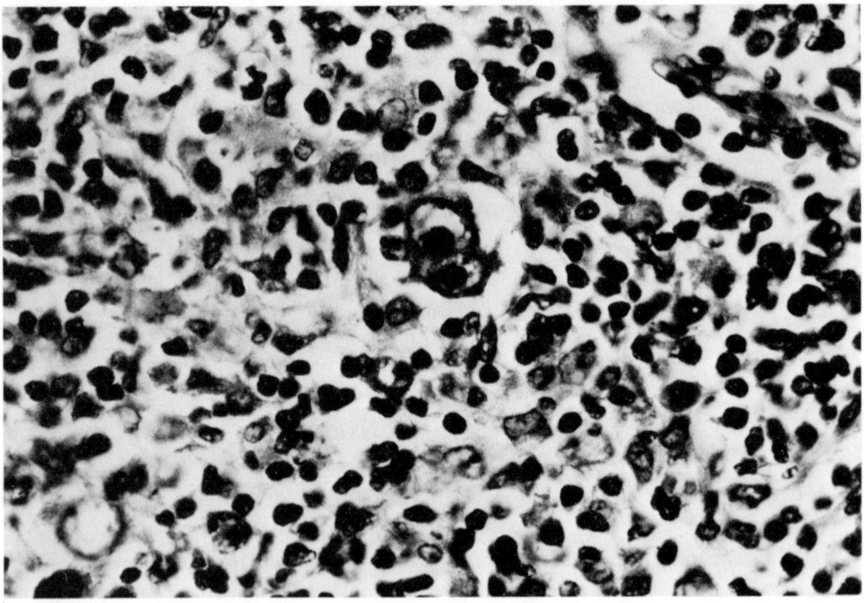

Figure 17: This high power photomicrograph shows a typical Reed-Sternberg cell, which is binucleate and has two prominent large nucleoli. There is perinucleolar clearing. The amount of cytoplasm is moderate.

disease have demonstrated that it spreads via lymphatic channels in a contiguous fashion from node group to node group. Involvement of spleen, liver, and bone marrow by Hodgkin's disease occurs by hematogeneous spread and indicates advanced disease. Contiguous extranodal organ invasion from adjacent nodal disease also occurs and has less grave prognostic implications.

Although Hodgkin's disease can occur at any age, there are bimodal incidence peaks in the third and fifth decades. The disease is more frequent in males. Younger patients tend to present with more localized disease, while older patients manifest more widespread disease.

Classification of Hodgkin's Disease

The standard classification of Hodgkin's disease is the Rye modification of the Lukes and Butler classification system as shown in Table 5. This classification of Hodgkin's disease is based upon the

Table 5
Classification of Hodgkin's Disease

Rye Modification		*Lukes and Butler Classification*
Lymphocyte predominance	→	Lymphocytic and histiocytic, nodular
	→	Lymphocytic and histiocytic, diffuse
Nodular sclerosis	→	Nodular sclerosis
Mixed cellularity	→	Mixed
Lymphocyte depletion	→	Diffuse fibrosis
	→	Reticular

relative number and type of RS cells and RS variants, the presence or absence (and type) of collagen, and the relative frequency of lymphocytes.

Lymphocyte Predominance Hodgkin's Disease (LPHD)

LPHD can have either a macronodular or a diffuse pattern of nodal infiltration. The predominant cell is the small round lymphocyte. Scattered histiocytes, sometimes in clusters, may also be seen. A distinctive RS cell variant called the L and H cell is present. This has a large, lobulated to polypoid nucleus with fine chromatin, inconspicuous nucleoli, and moderate to abundant pale cytoplasm (Fig. 18). Diagnostic RS cells are quite rare, as are other cells such as eosinophils and plasma cells. Necrosis and fibrosis are not seen.

Nodular Sclerosis Hodgkin's Disease (NSHD)

In NSHD, well-formed birefringent collagen bands arise from a thickened capsule and separate the Hodgkin's disease into large lobules (Figs. 19, 20). A distinctive RS cell variant called the lacunar cell is present. This has a small, hyperlobated to vesicular nucleus, variably prominent nucleoli, and a moderate amount of water-clear cytoplasm that retracts from surrounding cells during formalin fixation, creating a lacunar space (Fig. 20). The number of lacunar cells and diagnostic RS cells varies, and in some cases the lacunar cells may predominate. Other cell types such as lymphocytes, eosinophils, and plasma cells are fairly common. Necrosis is frequent.

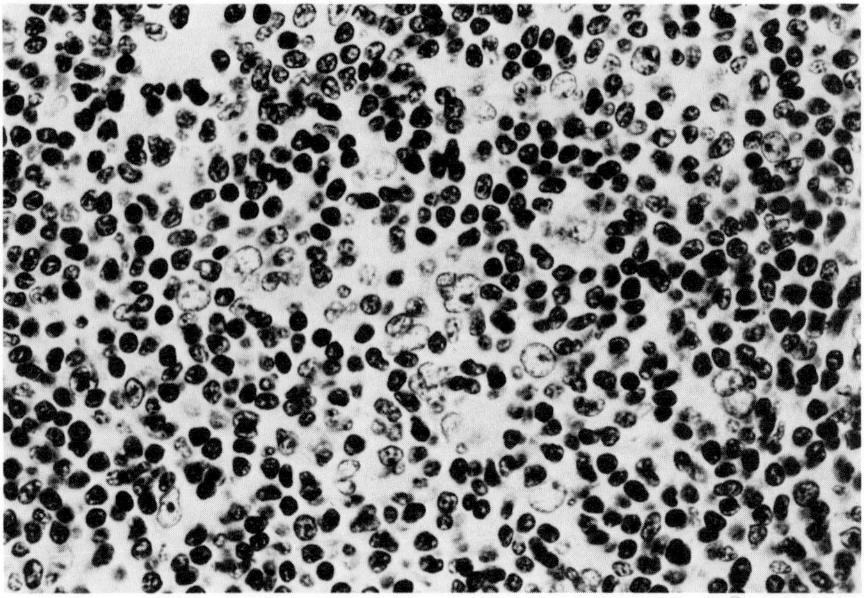

Figure 18: This high power photomicrograph of lymphocyte predominance Hodgkin's disease contains numerous round, mature-appearing lymphocytes. In addition, L and H type Reed-Sternberg cells are identified. These cells have polypoid vesicular nuclei and variably prominent nucleoli.

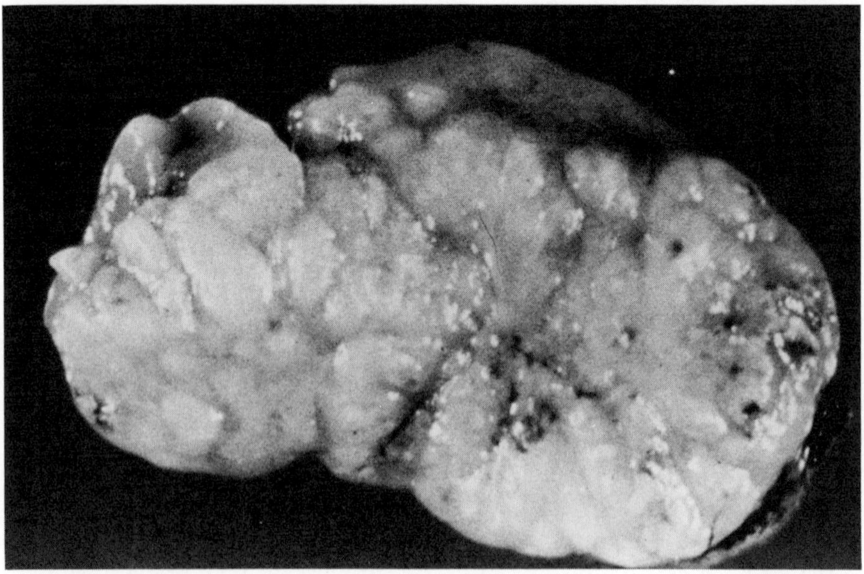

Figure 19: This gross photograph of nodular sclerosis Hodgkin's disease shows the variably sized nodules created by the fibrous bands.

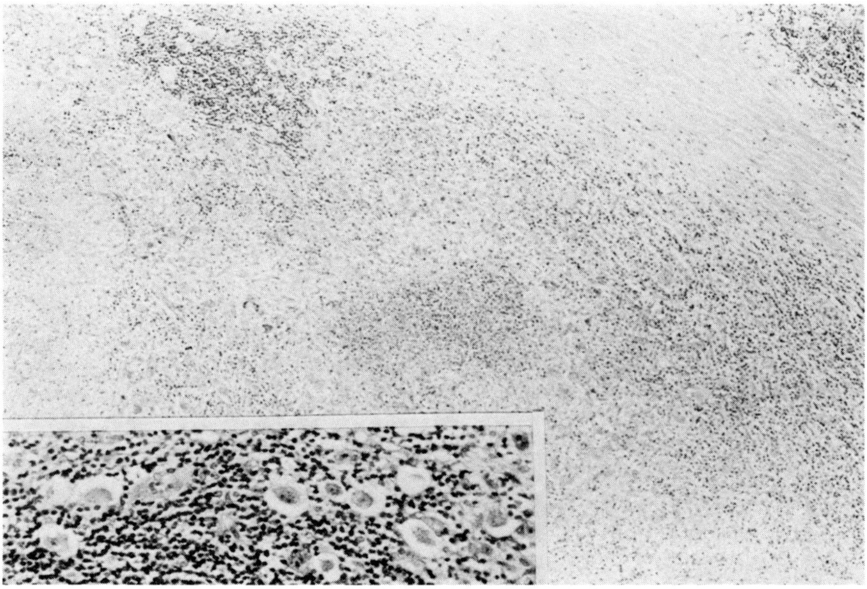

Figure 20: This medium power photomicrograph of nodular sclerosis Hodgkin's disease shows a wide collagen band and an adjacent infiltrate in which large and small cells are evident. A focus on central necrosis is present. *Inset:* high power magnification of this infiltrate shows large cells with the typical features of lacunar cells in which prominent cytoplasmic retraction is seen.

Mixed Cellularity Hodgkin's Disease (MCHD)

Those cases of Hodgkin's disease that do not readily fit into the three other groups are called MCHD. Diagnostic RS cells are readily identifiable (Fig. 21). The mixed cell population usually contains many eosinophils and a fair number of plasma cells and lymphocytes. Necrosis is fairly common.

Lymphocyte Depletion Hodgkin's Disease (LDHD)

There are two types of LDHD: reticular and diffuse fibrosis. In the reticular type, RS cells and RS variants are quite numerous while other cell types are disproportionately decreased. Sarcomatous RS cells may be seen (Fig. 22). These cells exhibit a wide range of bizarre

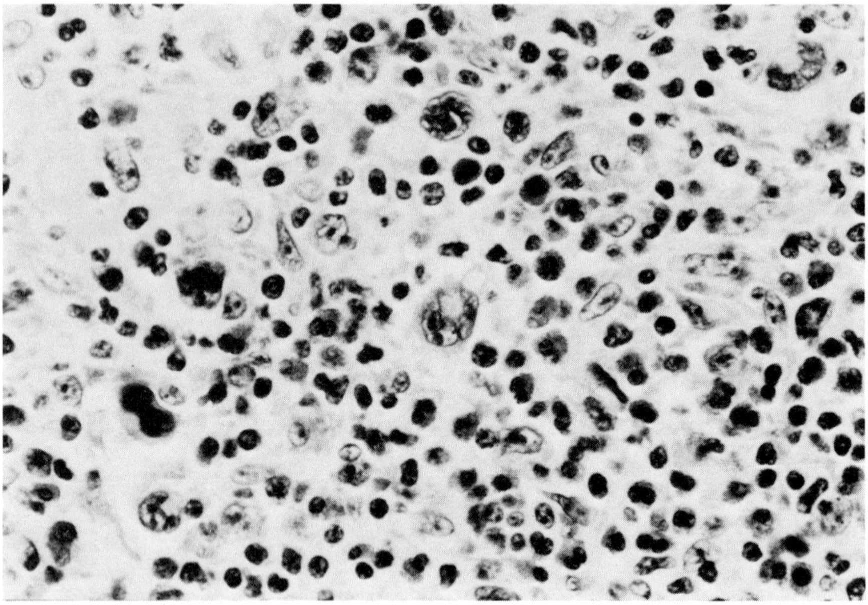

Figure 21: This high power photomicrograph of mixed cellularity Hodgkin's disease shows multiple cell types including lymphocytes, neutrophils, plasma cells, and large binucleate and multinucleated Reed-Sternberg cells.

configurations, some being huge and having giant nucleoli. In the diffuse fibrosis type, there are large acellular areas in which there is disorganized, non-birefringent collagen. Scattered RS cells and variants are present and other cell types are decreased. Necrosis is variable.

Relative Frequencies of Hodgkin's Disease in Adults and Children

Hodgkin's disease is more common in adults than in children. Although percentages between series vary, the more frequent types of Hodgkin's disease in adults are NSHD and MCHD, with NSHD usually being the most common (70% in some series). LPHD and LDHD are both uncommon in the United States. Hodgkin's disease is less common in children than in adults, but the distribution of histological types does not differ greatly except for the rarity of LDHD in children.

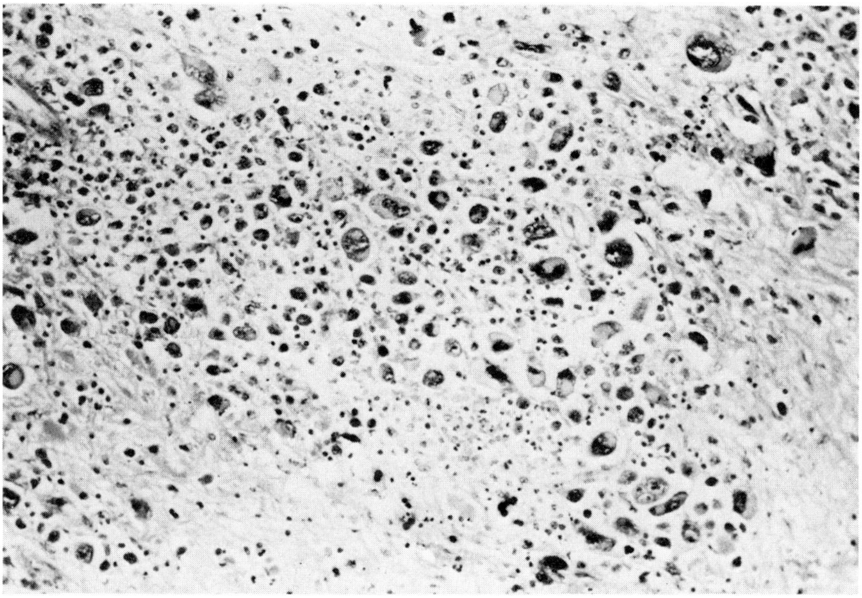

Figure 22: This medium power photomicrograph of lymphocyte depletion Hodgkin's disease shows numerous atypical Reed-Sternberg cells and Reed-Sternberg variants. Other cell types are disproportionately depleted.

Diagnosis of Hodgkin's Disease in Spleen, Liver, and Bone Marrow

The diagnosis of Hodgkin's disease in extranodal sites such as spleen, liver, and bone marrow is essential for accurate staging. The criteria for the diagnosis of Hodgkin's disease in these sites is the same for all morphological subtypes. The requirements for an extranodal diagnosis of Hodgkin's disease vary, depending on whether there is a prior diagnosis of Hodgkin's disease in a lymph node. If the patient has no prior diagnosis of Hodgkin's disease in a lymph node, then the same stringent criteria for Hodgkin's disease diagnosis described above must be met within any extranodal site. Thus, diagnostic RS cells must be identified in the typical polycellular background of Hodgkin's disease before this diagnosis can be made. However, if the patient has a bonafide lymph node diagnosis of Hodgkin's disease, then involvement in extranodal sites can be diagnosed if one can find a discrete lesion comprised of atypical mononuclear cells with prominent nucleoli intermixed with lymphocytes, plasma cells, histiocytes, and/or eosinophils. In this circumstance, classic Reed-Sternberg cells are not necessary for the diagnosis.

Splenic involvement has been identified in up to 40% of patients with Hodgkin's disease who undergo staging laparotomy with splenectomy. The earliest infiltrates are localized to the periarteriolar lymphoid sheath of the white pulp. These can be quite small and difficult to identify by gross examination. However, there is a propensity for bulky mass formation by Hodgkin's disease in the spleen with large areas of architectural disruption (Fig. 23 A, B). The cellular infiltrates show admixed atypical mononuclear or binucleate RS cells and RS variants, together with the other cells typically seen. The earliest infiltrates in the liver are localized to the portal tracts, similar to most other types of malignant lymphoma. The cell types seen are similar to those in the spleen. Hepatic involvement is relatively infrequent and is always seen in conjunction with splenic involvement.

Bone marrow involvement is fairly uncommon at presentation. Rarely bone narrow involvement may be seen as a consequence of direct spread from nearby involved lymph nodes. However, most cases of bone marrow Hodgkin's disease are the result of hematogenous spread to random foci within the marrow. This type of hematogenous spread to bone marrow is virtually always associated with splenic involvement. When present, bone marrow Hodgkin's disease tends to form relatively large diffuse areas of architectural obliteration that are almost always associated with fibrosis. The cellularity of these areas varies from markedly hypercellular to markedly hypocellular, with extensive fibrosis. As emphasized for spleen and liver, atypical mononuclear cells within the typical cellular background must be seen before a diagnosis can be made, assuming there is a prior lymph node diagnosis of Hodgkin's disease. Most cases of bone marrow Hodgkin's disease occur in patients with NSHD and MCHD, although this is relatively more common in the rarer LDHD.

Extranodal Lymphoma and Pseudolymphoma

Introduction

There are two types of extranodal lymphoma, one of which manifests with extranodal disease and is essentially localized to this site. In the other, there is widespread nodal involvement together with

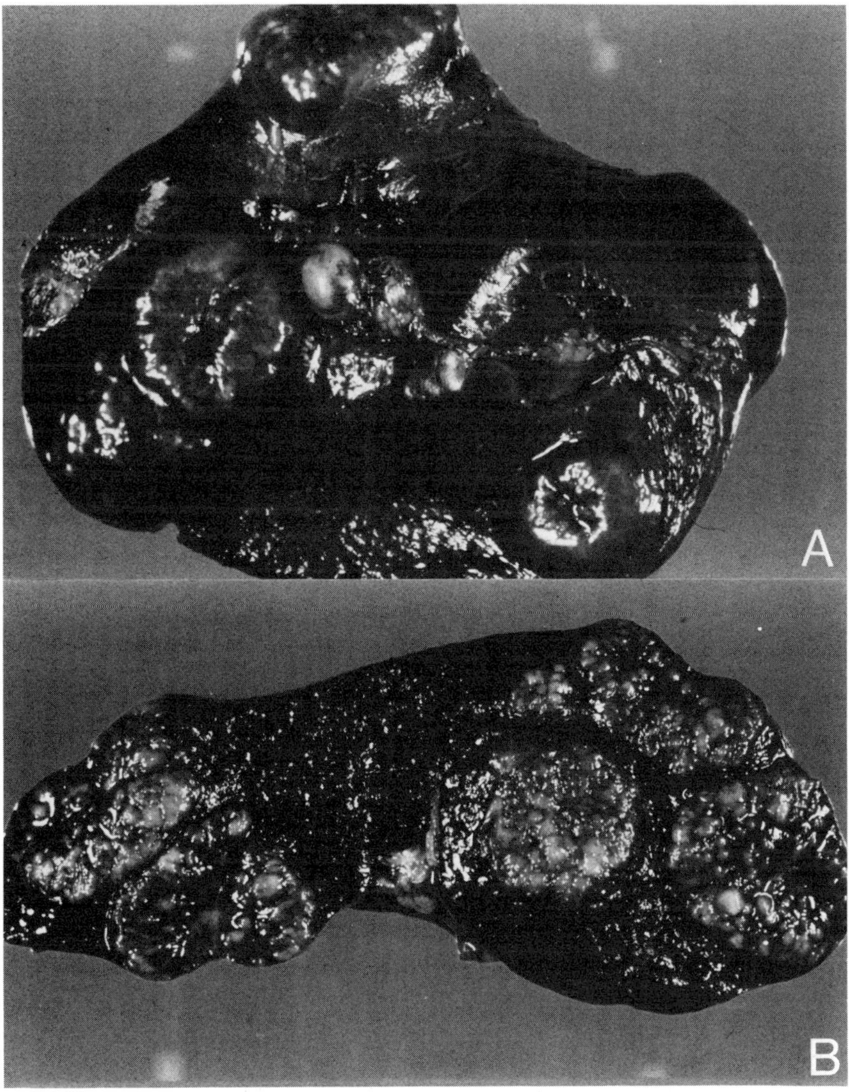

Figure 23: (A) This gross photograph of the external surface of a spleen involved by Hodgkin's disease shows multiple discrete mass lesions that project from the capsular surface. In addition, the lymph nodes at the splenic hilum, shown in the center of the field, are also enlarged, indicative of lymphoma. (B) On cut-section, this spleen shows multiple discrete mass lesions.

concurrent significant extranodal disease. The frequency of extranodal lymphoma varies according to how the disease is defined. Exclusive extranodal lymphoma constitutes about 10–25% of all NHL. All patients with significant extranodal manifestations, with or without concurrent lymph node disease, represent 20–50% of all NHL. Although patients with Hodgkin's disease can have extranodal spread, especially to sites adjacent to nodal disease, this phenomenon is relatively rare and usually does not dominate the clinical course. Localized extranodal Hodgkin's disease is uncommon and consequently the discussion of extranodal lymphoma will be largely limited to NHL, with only occasional mention of Hodgkin's disease.

The head and neck region and GI tract are the most common sites of extranodal lymphoma in most series. Extranodal NHL is also seen with relative frequency in lung, skin, thyroid, testes, breast, bone, and CNS. The most common morphological cell types comprising extranodal NHL are poorly differentiated lymphocytic lymphoma, predominantly diffuse but occasionally nodular, as well as diffuse histiocytic lymphoma. In addition, undifferentiated and well-differentiated lymphocytic lymphomas may present in extranodal sites, especially undifferentiated lymphoma. However, due to their rarity, they do not constitute a large fraction of extranodal lymphomas.

In all extranodal sites, one must distinguish malignant lymphoma from benign, variably atypical, lymphocytic, plasmacellular, and/or histiocytic proliferations, which are commonly called pseudolymphomas. This distinction is frequently quite challenging since there are many gross and microscopic similarities between malignant lymphoma and pseudolymphoma. Pseudolymphomas have been described in almost every site in which extranodal lymphomas have been reported to occur. In general, the pseudolymphomas have a variety of cell types, lack the marked atypia of lymphomas, and contain reactive germinal centers. Since individual pseudolymphomas may not exhibit all of these benign features, one must sometimes rely on immunological studies of the cells to distinguish benign from malignant lymphoreticular proliferations. Immunological studies would demonstrate a monoclonal (arising from a single parent clone) population of cells in lymphoma and a polyclonal (arising from multiple parent clones) population of cells in pseudolymphoma.

In addition, extranodal lymphomas must be distinguished from other malignancies, especially carcinomas. This can usually be accomplished by careful cytological evaluation of the cells in conjunction with histochemical studies such as mucin and glycogen stains. Electron microscopy may sometimes be necessary to distinguish lymphoma from poorly differentiated carcinoma.

Head and Neck

The orbit is a common site of head and neck lymphoma and pseudolymphoma and the two processes are clinically indistinguishable. By pathological examinations, most orbital lymphomas are diffuse PDLL, while WDLL and nodular PDLL are also seen with relative frequency. The pseudolymphomatous processes consist of inflammatory pseudotumor and various other reactive processes. The pseudolymphomas generally contain some germinal centers and frequently have admixed plasma cells.

Other sites of extranodal lymphoma of the head and neck are tonsil, parotid gland, and tongue. Although PDLL also predominates in these sites, diffuse histiocytic lymphoma (DHL) is relatively common. Thyroid lymphoma will be discussed later in this chapter.

Gastrointestinal Tract

Although lymphomas of the GI tract are a common type of extranodal lymphoma, they represent only 1% of all GI tract neoplasms. The stomach is the most frequent site of GI tract lymphoma (40–75%), although these lymphomas comprise less than 5% of all gastric malignancies. In order of decreasing frequency, the remaining sites of GI tract lymphoma are small bowel, ileocecal region, and large bowel. A small number of patients will have tumors in multiple sites.

Malignant lymphomas of the GI tract vary somewhat in gross appearance, depending upon their location. Those within the stomach frequently resemble carcinomas as the wall and rugal folds are thickened, and the mass may be ulcerated (Fig. 24). Occasional gastric lymphomas are polypoid. In the small bowel, malignant lymphomas tend to have intact overlying mucosa, although focal ulceration may be seen. These small bowel lymphomas have an annular, nodular, or polypoid gross appearance. Malignant lymphoma of the large bowel is quite rare and comprises less than 1% of colonic malignancies. Although gross descriptions are scant, large bowel lymphomas are usually well circumscribed and may be variably polypoid, predominantly intramural, or project outward from the serosa (Fig. 25).

The most common morphological type of GI tract NHL is DHL (60–80%) (Fig. 26). Some authors suggest that these large cell lymphomas are actually derived from true histiocytes, but most others suggest that the majority of GI tract lymphomas are derived from transformed B lymphocytes. Large cell lymphomas comprised of im-

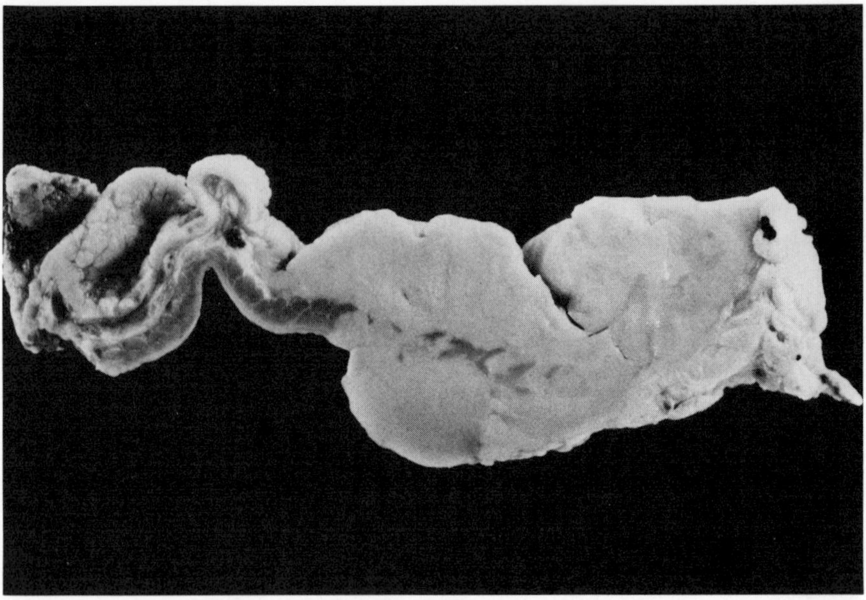

Figure 24: This gross photograph of a gastric lymphoma on cut-section shows a transmural lymphomatous infiltrate. The intact gastric mucosa and muscular wall is evident in the left half of the photograph. The lymphoma obliterates all normal architectural structures except for small islands of residual smooth muscle. The lymphoma has a characteristic homogeneous fish-flesh appearance.

munoblasts predominate in some studies. Other morphological types of GI tract lymphoma include WDLL, PDLL, mixed lymphocytic-histiocytic lymphomas, and undifferentiated lymphoma. The pattern of infiltration is more frequently diffuse than nodular for all cell types. Undifferentiated lymphomas are more common in young patients and tend to involve the ileocecal region (see Fig. 15). Prognosis is better for patients with localized disease and favorable histology such as WDLL. Hodgkin's disease very rarely presents with GI tract manifestations.

Various pseudolymphomatous infiltrates have also been described in the GI tract, but these disorders are less common than lymphomas. Although the stomach is the most common site for GI tract "pseudolymphomas," they can occur in any region (Fig. 27). Gastric pseudolymphomas (also called lymphoid hyperplasia) are frequently associated with peptic ulcer disease. Pseudolymphomas are relatively

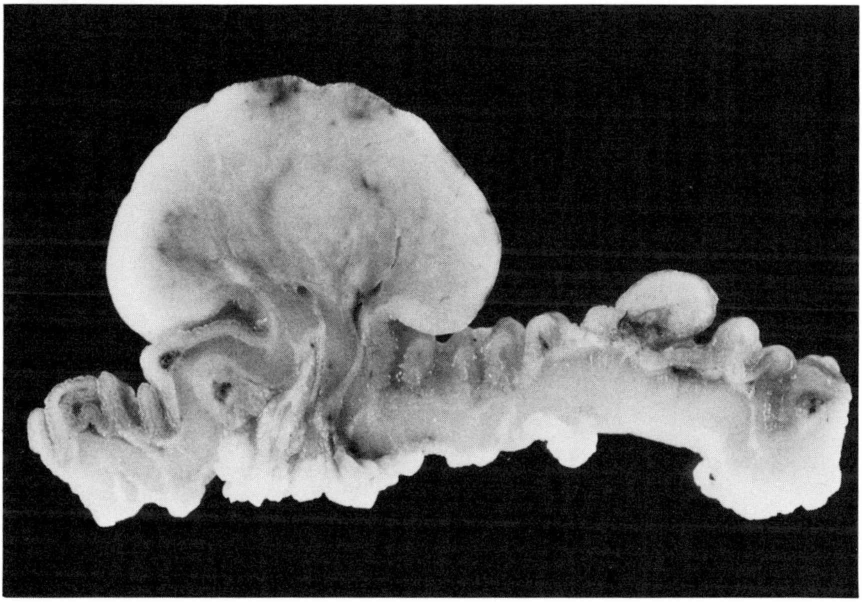

Figure 25: This rectal lymphoma has a distinctly polypoid appearance.

common in the rectum and distinctly uncommon in the small bowel, and they tend to have a polypoid or nodular gross appearance. Some helpful morphological features used to distinguish benign lymphoid infiltrates from NHL include a polymorphous cellular infiltrate, lack of significant cytological atypia, and the presence of germinal centers in lymphoid hyperplasia (pseudolymphoma) (Fig. 28). These features are generally absent in NHL. As in other sites, immunological evaluation may be necessary to distinguish lymphoma from pseudolymphoma.

Lung

Both lymphomas and pseudolymphomas of the lung are rare, and the incidence is minute in comparison with epithelial tumors of the lung. Most cases of lymphoma in the lung represent secondary disease in patients with previously diagnosed nodal lymphoma. In this circumstance, there are about equal numbers of cases of Hodgkin's disease and NHL. The lung is the only extranodal site in which Hodgkin's disease is seen with any frequency. Pulmonary Hodgkin's disease

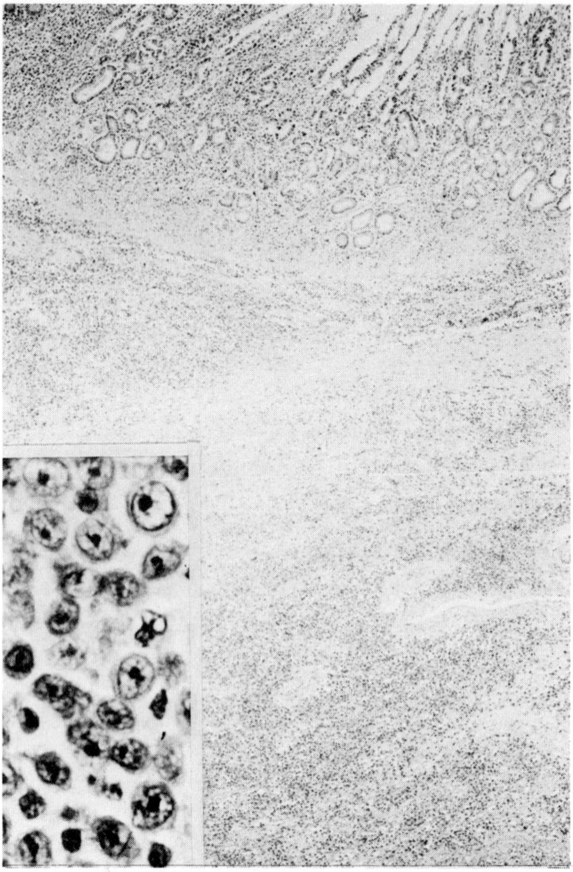

Figure 26: This low power photomicrograph of a gastric diffuse histiocytic lymphoma shows infiltration of all layers by the lymphoma. *Inset:* The cytologic features of these cells are illustrated. The lymphoma cells have generally round nuclear contours and minimal to moderate amounts of cytoplasm.

is virtually always associated with mediastinal involvement. NHL can present with isolated pulmonary disease and most of these cases are histiocytic (large cell) lymphomas. Malignant lymphomas of the lung are usually solid, firm masses of variable size, although occasional cystic areas result from necrosis, especially in histiocytic (large cell) lymphomas and Hodgkin's disease. Adjacent lymph nodes may be involved in NHL, and are virtually always involved in Hodgkin's disease.

A variety of pulmonary pseudolymphomatous processes, including pulmonary angiitis and granulomatosis, as well as lymphomatoid

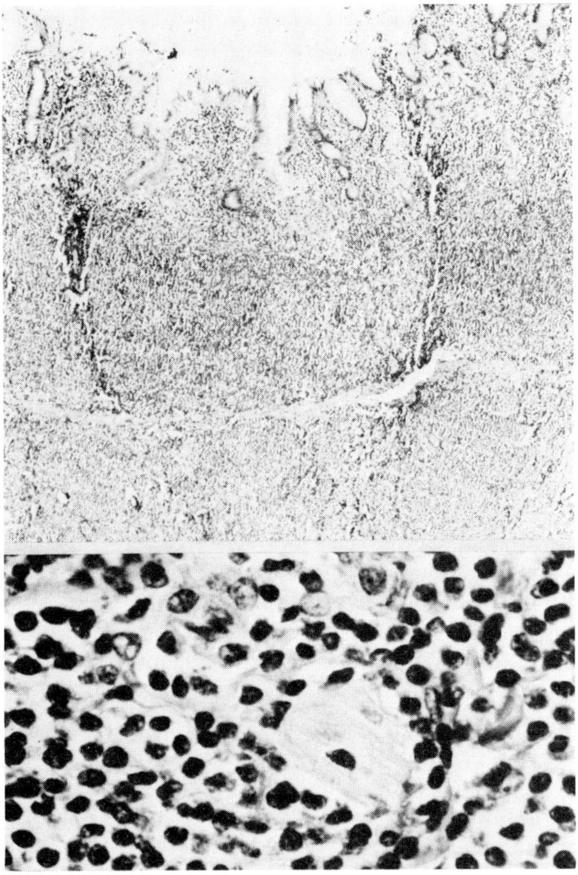

Figure 27: This low power photomicrograph of gastric pseudolymphoma (lymphoid hyperplasia) shows predominant involvement of the mucosa and submucosa. The lymphocytes do not extend through the muscular wall. *Inset:* The cells comprising this infiltrate consist predominantly of small, round, mature-appearing lymphocytes.

granulomatosis, may be difficult to distinguish from lymphoma. In fact, these processes appear morphologically and clinically to merge into malignant lymphoma. In general, these pseudolymphomatous processes exhibit a polymorphous cell population with variable numbers (usually low) of atypical cells. Those cases with a predominance of atypical cells are thought to represent the evolution of malignant lymphoma within the underlying process. Specific anatomical structures within the lung, such as vessels or bronchi, can show widespread selective involvement in the early stages of these disorders. A spectrum

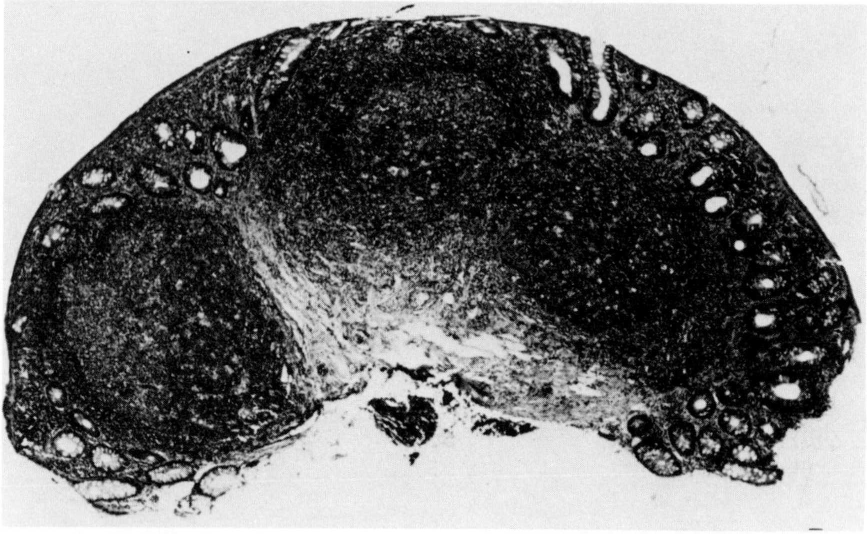

Figure 28: This low power photomicrograph of lymphoid hyperplasia of the rectum shows three prominent, distinct germinal centers.

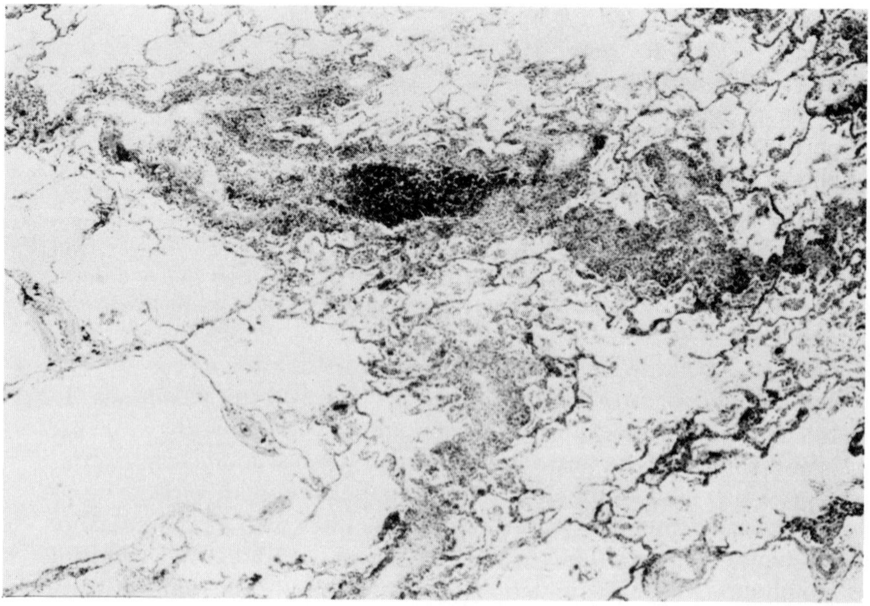

Figure 29: This low power photomicrograph of lung shows a distinctly angiocentric infiltrative process. The cells percolate through all layers of the vessel wall.

of angiocentric pulmonary disorders have been described (Fig. 29). In all types there is vascular infiltration by a variety of cell types that may be associated with necrosis and granuloma formation. In one type, Wegener's granulomatosis, the infiltrate consists of lymphocytes, plasma cells, and eosinophils. Discrete granulomata are fairly common. In another type of angiitis, lymphomatoid granulomatosis, atypical lymphoid cells are present and can even predominate. Mitotic activity increases with the number of atypical cells. Bronchocentric pulmonary granulomatous infiltrates have also been described, but these are not as numerous as the angiocentric processes.

Localized pulmonary pseudolymphomas with formation of a single mass lesion, characterized by the same cell types seen in pseudolymphomas from other sites, have also been described. In these pseudolymphomas, multiple mature-appearing cell types and germinal centers are found.

Skin

Cutaneous NHL, excluding mycosis fungoides, can be localized to skin or can occur in conjunction with nodal disease (Fig. 30 A, B). The head and neck region are the most commonly involved sites and most cases have the morphological features of DHL.

Other morphological types seen with some frequency are lymphoblastic lymphoma, diffuse mixed lymphocytic-histiocytic lymphoma, and undifferentiated lymphoma. Although less common, WDLL and nodular PDLL have also been described in the skin. Survival is better for patients with disease confined to skin and with favorable histological subtypes (such as WDLL and nodular PDLL).

The distinction between cutaneous lymphoma and lymphoid hyperplasia can be extremely difficult. In general, the malignant lymphomas extend more deeply into the dermis and subcutaneous tissue and are composed of more monotonous and atypical cells (Fig. 31). In cutaneous lymphoid hyperplasia (pseudolymphoma), the infiltrate is not generally as extensive and multiple cell types and even germinal centers may be seen (Fig. 32).

Mycosis fungoides (MF) is a morphologically and clinically distinctive primary cutaneous extranodal lymphoma, which arises from postthymic, helper T lymphocytes. The earliest infiltrates of MF have a marked propensity for intraepidermal localization, while all other types of cutaneous lymphoma tend to involve deep dermis and subcutaneous tissue selectively (Fig. 33). The cells of MF vary in size and

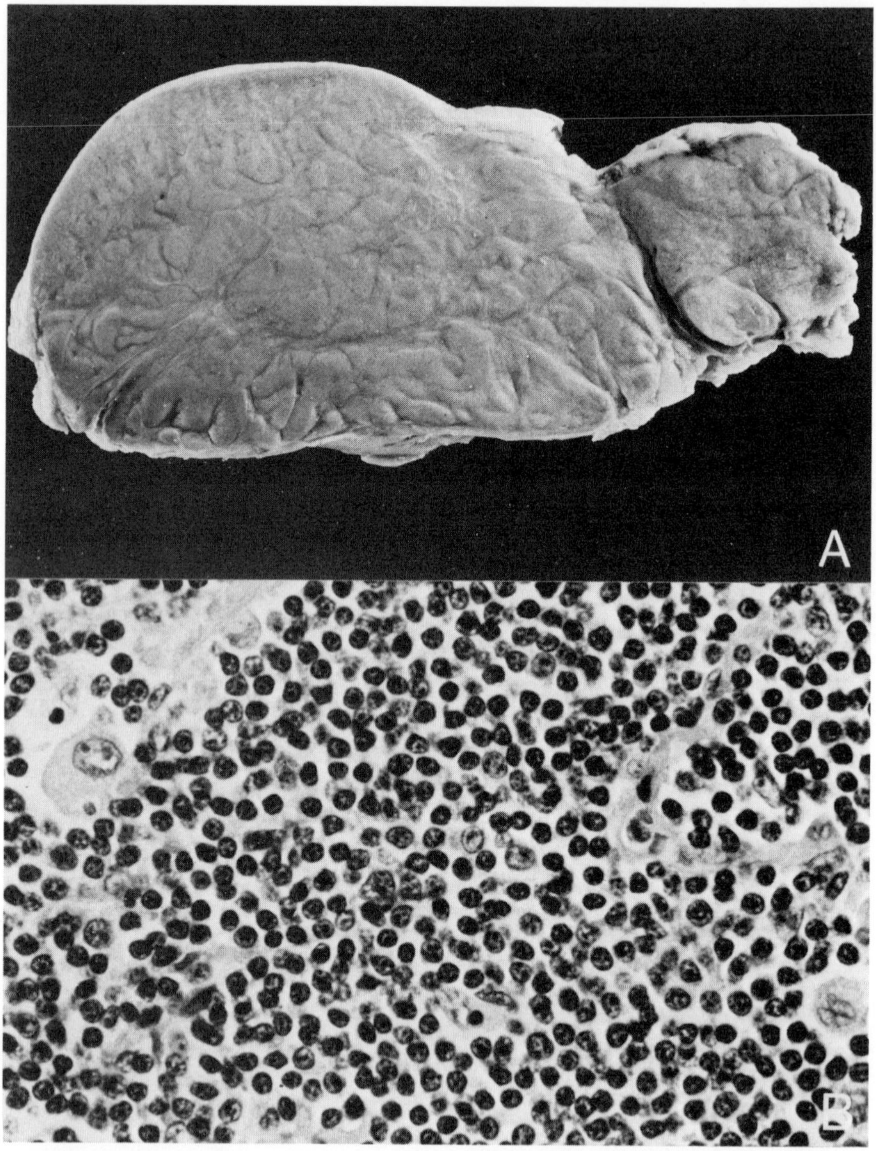

Figure 30: (A) This gross photograph of an extremely large cutaneous lymphoma shows a homogeneous mass without appreciable hemorrhage or necrosis. Collagen formation without the lymphoma accounts for the irregularly shaped nodules. Intact skin is present on the upper surface of this lymphoma. (B) High power photomicrograph of this cutaneous lymphoma shows a monotonous infiltrate of small round lymphocytes consistent with a diagnosis of WDLL. Note macrophage in upper left-hand corner for size comparison.

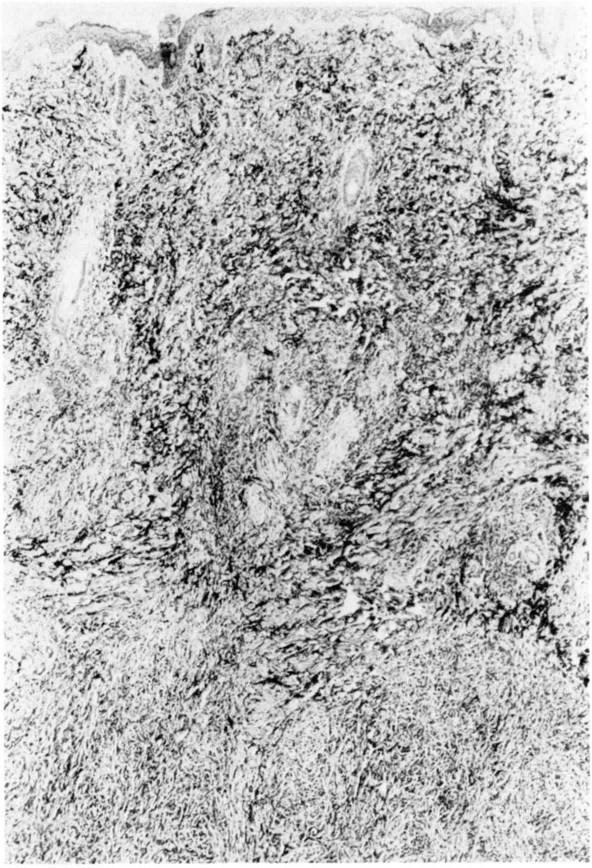

Figure 31: This low power photomicrograph of skin shows an extensive lymphomatous infiltrate involving the entire dermis with extension into the subcutaneous tissue. There is epidermal sparing by this lymphoma.

are characterized by extreme nuclear irregularity, giving the nuclei a cerebriform appearance. The nuclear chromatin is dense and nucleoli are inconspicuous. The amount of cytoplasm is variable. These MF cells are occasionally very large, but the majority are intermediately sized. MF is typically localized to skin for long periods before systemic spread, heralded by lymphadenopathy, occurs. Early involvement in lymph nodes selects the paracortical region of the node with sparing of the follicles. Circulating MF cells, also called Sezary cells, can be seen fairly early in the disease course and can actually precede bone marrow involvement (Fig. 33).

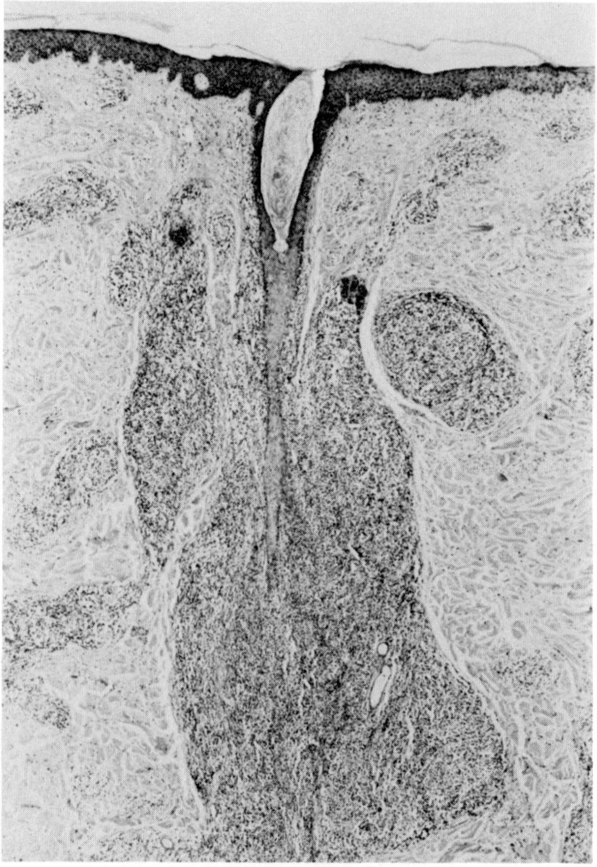

Figure 32: This low power photomicrograph of lymphoid hyperplasia of the skin shows relative preservation of normal anatomic structures and localized lymphoid infiltrates.

Testes

Although the testes can be the only site of NHL, testicular lymphoma is more commonly the site of an initial manifestation of more widespread disease. Even those patients with disease localized to the testes after adequate evaluation of other sites frequently manifest subsequent early widespread disease. Most cases of testicular lymphoma are DHL. PDLL, lymphoblastic lymphoma, and diffuse mixed lymphocytic-histiocytic lymphoma are seen less frequently. WDLL and Hodgkin's disease virtually never present as a testicular mass. Nodular lymphomas only rarely present with testicular involvement.

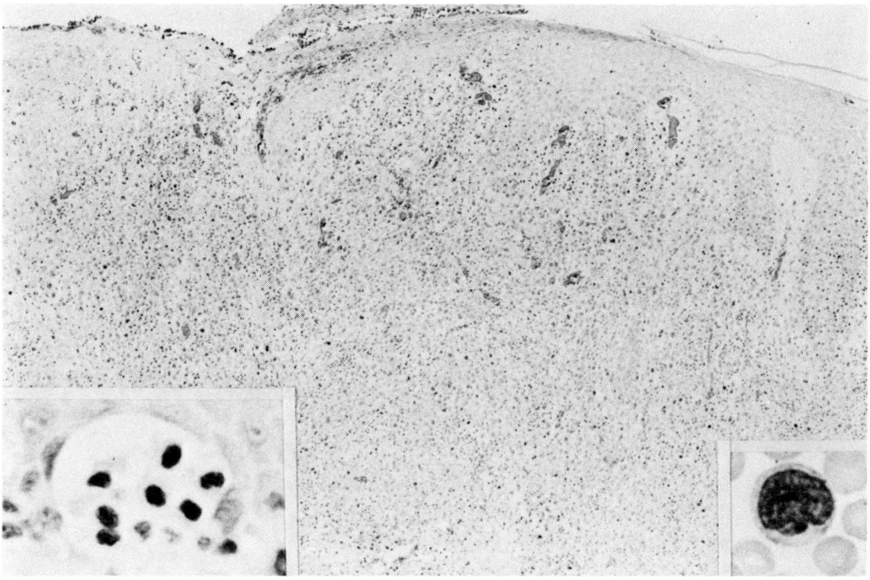

Figure 33: This low power photomicrograph of skin shows extensive infiltration by mycosis fungoides. These lymphoma cells are epidermotropic and also infiltrate the entire dermis. *Insets:* These show a Pautrier's microabscess at the dermal-epidermal junction and a circulating mycosis-Sezary cell in the blood. Marked nuclear irregularity is evident in this cell.

The lymphomatous infiltrates of all cytological types percolate diffusely within the interstitium which consequently expands greatly (Fig. 34). Seminiferous tubules are surrounded by the lymphoma and eventually obliterated. Occasional spared seminiferous tubules can be widely scattered within the lymphomatous infiltrate (Fig. 34). Pseudolymphomatous processes involving the testes have not been described, although orchitis secondary to various infections and inflammatory processes is well known.

Thyroid

The thyroid gland is a relatively uncommon site of extranodal lymphoma. Despite their relative rarity, the clinical and pathologic features of thyroid lymphomas have been fairly well described. This disease occurs almost exclusively in middle-aged to elderly patients and there is a striking female preponderance. There is very good evidence that these lymphomas do truly arise in the thyroid gland, and locally confined disease is common. Only one-fifth of patients have docu-

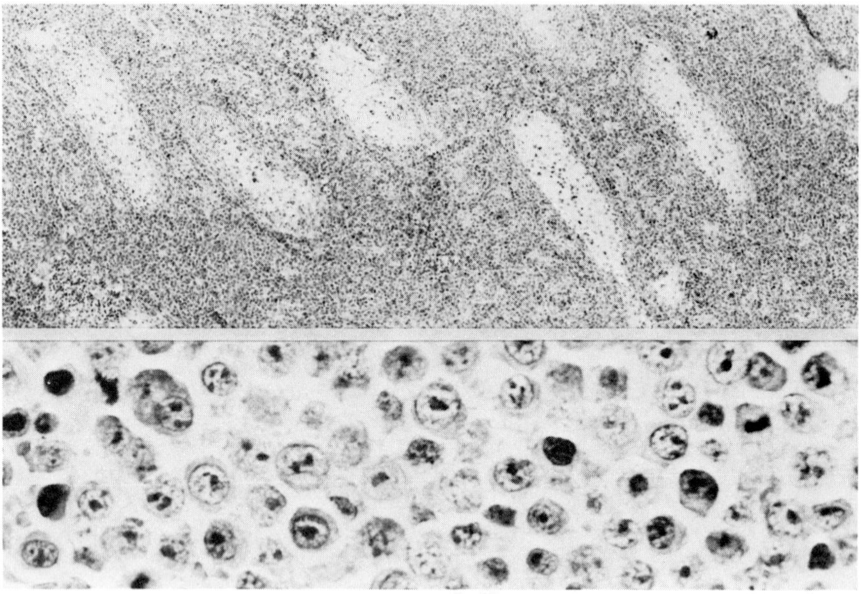

Figure 34: The upper part of this photomicrograph shows a medium power picture of lymphomatous infiltration of the testes. A few widely scattered residual seminiferous tubules are evident. The lower portion of this photomicrograph shows a high power view of the lymphoma cells. These cells are large in size, have round nuclear contours, and show focal plasmacytoid differentiation. Thus this diffuse histiocytic lymphoma appears to be comprised of immunoblasts.

mented cervical lymph node involvement. Although reported incidences vary, there tends to be a high frequency of DHL in thyroid extranodal lymphomas. Other cell types described are nodular histiocytic lymphoma, PDLL (usually diffuse, but also nodular), lymphomas with plasmacytoid differentiation, and true plasmacytomas. Nodular lymphomas account for about 10% of cases of thyroid NHL. Histological types reported only rarely include WDLL and undifferentiated lymphoma. Infrequent cases of Hodgkin's disease of the thyroid have been reported. There is a very strong association of thyroid lymphoma with an underlying lymphocytic thyroiditis, and several authors have suggested that a malignant clone arises out of the lymphocytic thyroiditis. Because of this frequent association, it can sometimes be difficult to distinguish one from the other. Lymphocytic thyroiditis shows a variable extent of cellular infiltration, consists predominantly of mature, small round lymphocytes, may contain germinal centers, and does not usually efface the normal architecture (Fig. 35). These benign cells can, however, penetrate the fibrous capsule of the thyroid gland. Malignant lymphomas are distinguishable from thyroiditis by the presence of cytological atypia and immaturity as well as architectural effacement. Features of thyroid lymphomas that are associated with an unfavorable prognosis include necrosis, capsular invasion, a diffuse pattern of infiltration, and involvement of cervical lymph nodes.

Bone

Malignant lymphoma of bone, which accounts for about 5% of extranodal lymphomas, is generally a manifestation of widespread disease, and patients with disease confined to bone are rare. Although a variety of histological types have been described, DHL usually predominates (50–60% of cases). Other histological types seen with relative frequency are diffuse mixed lymphocytic-histiocytic lymphoma

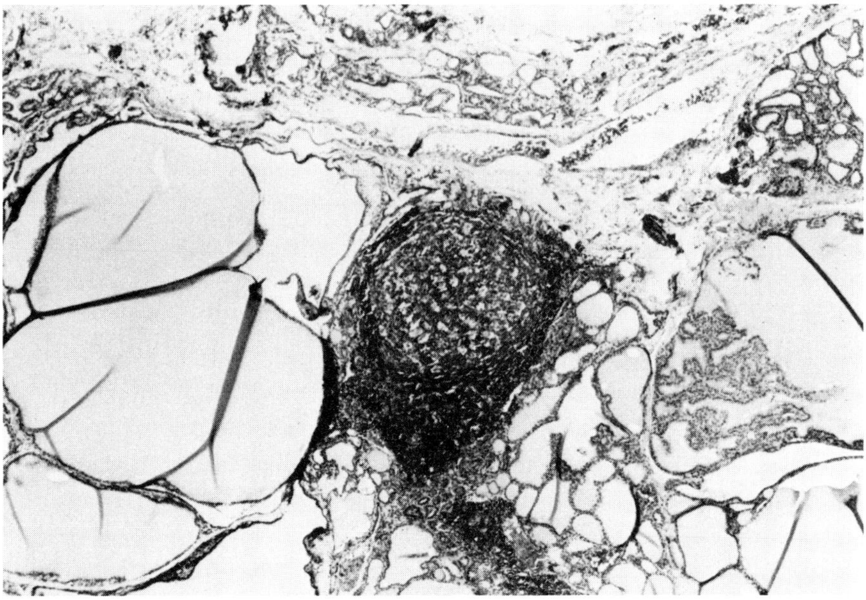

Figure 35: This photomicrograph of lymphocytic thyroiditis shows a prominent reactive follicle with a large germinal center surrounded by thyroid follicles.

and diffuse PDLL. Fibrosis and necrosis are common. Occasional patients with Hodgkin's disease will have radiographically apparent bone infiltration immediately adjacent to sites of nodal disease.

Pseudolymphomatous infiltrates of the bone have not been described, and the most likely disease to enter into the differential of primary bone lymphoma is Ewing's sarcoma. This can be distinguished from lymphoma by the relatively small size of the sarcoma cells and the abundant cytoplasmic glycogen. Because of their cell junctions, Ewing's sarcoma cells form cell clusters on imprint preparations and bone marrow aspirate smears, while lymphoma cells, which lack cell junctions, do not cluster on these preparations (Fig. 36).

Central Nervous System (CNS)

Primary CNS lymphoma, an uncommon site of extranodal lymphoma, has been noted with increased frequency in renal transplant

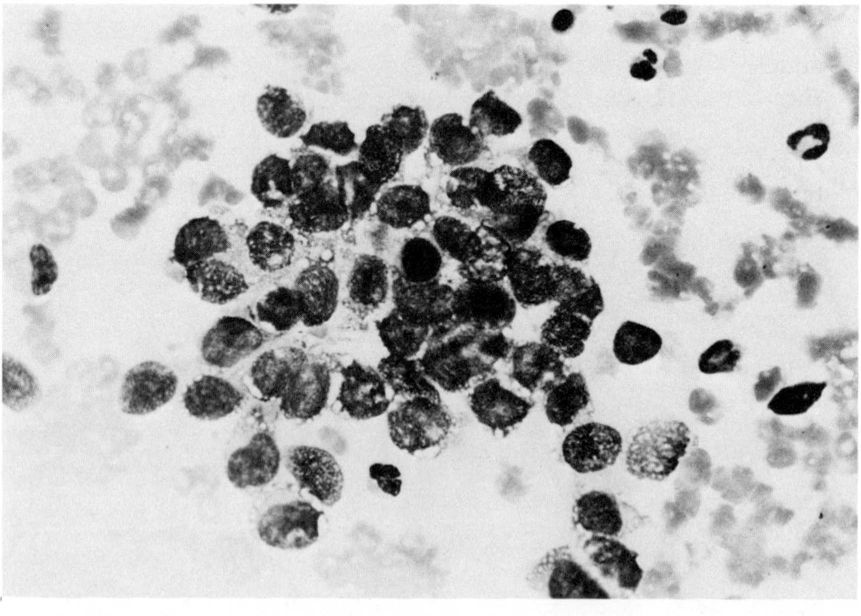

Figure 36: This bone marrow aspirate smear shows an aggregate of metastatic Ewing's sarcoma cells. The clumping is attributed to the cytoplasmic junctions of the cells. These tumor cells also have prominent cytoplasmic vacuoles that contain glycogen.

patients. Most cases are DHL (about 60%), and the only other common histological type is PDLL. Although the lymphoma cells can sometimes be identified in the cerebrospinal fluid (CSF), brain biopsy is usually necessary to establish the diagnosis. In contrast with many of the other extranodal lymphomas, primary CNS lymphoma is typically localized. Except for benign true histiocytic proliferations, pseudolymphomas have not been well described in the CNS.

Breast

Both lymphoma and pseudolymphoma of the breast are extremely uncommon lesions representing well under 1% of breast neoplasms. Primary lymphoma of the breast is virtually always diffuse and most cases are undifferentiated lymphoma. The next most common group is DHL; rare cases of lymphoblastic lymphoma arising in the breast have been reported. The lymphomatous infiltrates percolate around preexisting structures, but architectural obliteration eventually occurs. The lymphoma cells are atypical and immature.

Pseudolymphoma, in contrast with lymphoma, has a distinctly nodular microscopic appearance, which is commonly due to the presence of germinal centers, and does not show cytological atypia or immaturity. Patients with pseudolymphoma of the breast often give a history of trauma to the site and it may represent an overwhelming response to injury.

Selected Reading

Berard, C., O'Connor, G.T., Thomas, L.B., et al.: Histopathological definition of Burkitt's tumor. *Bull. WHO* 40:601–607, 1969.

Burke, J.S., Butler, J.J., Fuller, L.M.: Malignant lymphomas of the thyroid: A clinicopathological study of 35 patients including ultrastructural observations. *Cancer* 39:1587–1602, 1977.

Butler, J.J.: The natural history of Hodgkin's disease and its classification, in Rebuck, J.W., Berard, C.W., Abell, M.R. (eds.): *The Reticuloendothelial System*. Baltimore, Williams & Wilkins, 1975, pp. 184–212.

Brunning, R.D., McKenna, R.W.: Bone marrow manifestations of malignant lymphoma and lymphoma-like conditions. *Pathol. Ann.* 14:1–59, 1979.

Burke, J.S., Hoppe, R.T., Cibull, M.L., et al.: Cutaneous malignant lymphoma: A pathologic study of 50 cases with clinical analysis of 37. *Cancer* 47:300–310, 1981.

Compagno, J., Oertel, J.E.: Malignant lymphoma and other lymphoproliferative disorders of the thyroid gland: A clinicopathological study of 245 cases. *Am. J. Clin. Pathol.* 74:1–11, 1980.

Evans, H.L., Winkelmann, R.K., Banks, P.M.: Differential diagnosis of malignant and benign cutaneous lymphoid infiltrates: A study of 57 cases in which malignant lymphoma had been diagnosed or suspected in the skin. *Cancer* 44:699–717, 1979.

Foucar, K., Armitage, J.O., Dick, F.R.: Malignant lymphoma, diffuse mixed small and large cell: A clinicopathological study of 47 cases. *Cancer* 51:2090–2099, 1983.

Foucar, K., McKenna, R.W., Frizzera, G., et al.: Incidence and patterns of bone marrow and blood involvement by lymphoma in relationship to the Lukes-Collins classification. *Blood* 54:1417–1422, 1979.

Jones, S.E., Fuks, Z., Bull, M., et al.: Non-Hodgkin's lymphomas. IV. Clinicopathological correlation in 405 cases. *Cancer* 31:806–823, 1973.

Kaplan, H.S.: Hodgkin's disease: Unfolding concepts concerning its nature, management and prognosis. *Cancer* 45:2439–2474, 1980.

Knowles, D.M., Jakobiec, F.A.: Ocular adnexal lymphoid neoplasms: Clinical, histopathologic, electron microscopic, and immunological characteristics. *Hum. Pathol.* 13:148–162, 1982.

Lewin, K.J., Ranchod, M., Dorfman, R.F.: Lymphomas of the gastrointestinal tract: A study of 117 cases presenting with gastrointestinal disease. *Cancer* 42:693–707, 1978.

Lukes, R.J.: Criteria for involvement of lymph node, bone marrow, spleen, and liver in Hodgkin's disease. *Cancer Res.* 31:1755–1764, 1971.

Lukes, R.J., Collins, R.D.: Immunological characterization of human malignant lymphomas. *Cancer* 34:1488–1503, 1974.

Mann, R.B., Jaffe, E.S., Berard, C.W.: Malignant lymphomas–a conceptual understanding of morphologic diversity. *Am. J. Pathol.* 94:105–175, 1979.

Nathwani, B.N.: A critical analysis of the classifications of non-Hodgkin's lymphomas. *Cancer* 44:347–384, 1979.

Nathwani, B.N., Diamond, L.W., Winberg, C.D., et al.: Lymphoblastic lymphoma: A clinicopathologic study of 95 patients. *Cancer* 48:2347–2357, 1981.

O'Carroll, D.I., McKenna, R.W., Brunning, R.D.: Bone marrow manifestations of Hodgkin's disease. *Cancer* 38:1717–1728, 1976.

Ranchod, M., Lewin, K.J., Dorfman, R.F.: Lymphoid hyperplasia of the gastrointestinal tract: A study of 26 cases and review of the literature. *Am. J. Surg. Pathol.* 2:383–400, 1978.

Rappaport, H.: *Tumors of the Hematopoietic System.* Washington, D.C., Armed Forces Institute of Pathology, 1966.

Risdall, R., Hoppe, R.T., Warnke, R.: Non-Hodgkin's lymphoma–a study of the evolution of the disease based upon 92 autopsied cases. *Cancer* 44:529–542, 1979.

Rudders, R.A., Ross, M.E., DeLellis, R.A.: Primary extranodal lymphoma–response to treatment and factors influencing prognosis. *Cancer* 42:406–416, 1978.

Saldana, M.J., Patchefsky, A.S., Israel, H.I., et al.: Pulmonary angiitis and granulomatosis–The relationship between histological features, organ involvement, and response to treatment. *Hum. Pathol.* 8:391–409, 1977.

Saltzstein, S.L.: Extranodal malignant lymphomas and pseudolymphomas. *Pathol. Ann.* 4:159–184, 1969.

Taylor, C.R., Russell, R., Lukes, R.J., et al.: An immunohistological study of immunoglobulin content of primary central nervous system lymphomas. *Cancer* 41:2197–2205, 1978.

The non-Hodgkin's lymphoma pathologic classification project: National Cancer Institute sponsored study of classifications of non-Hodgkin's lymphomas–Summary and description of a working formulation for clinical usage. *Cancer* 49:2112–2135, 1982.

Turner, R.R., Colby, T.V., MacKintosh, F.R.: Testicular lymphomas: A clinicopathologic study of 35 cases. *Cancer* 48:2095–2102, 1981.

Van Den Tweel, J.G., Lukes, R.J., Taylor, C.R.: Pathophysiology of lymphocyte transformation: A study of so-called composite lymphomas. *Am. J. Clin. Pathol.* 71:509–520, 1979.

Waldron, J.A., Leech, J.H., Glick, A.D., et al.: Malignant lymphoma of peripheral T-lymphocyte origin. *Cancer* 40:1604–1617, 1977.

Weingrad, D.N., Decosse, J.J., Sherlock, P., et al.: Primary gastrointestinal lymphoma: A 30-year review. *Cancer* 49:1258–1265, 1982.

Weisenburger, D.D., Nathwani, B.N., Diamond, L.W., et al.: Malignant lymphoma, intermediate lymphocytic type: A clinicopathologic study of 42 cases. *Cancer* 48:1415–1425, 1981.

Wright, D.H.: Burkitt's lymphoma: A review of the pathology, immunology, and possible etiologic factors. *Pathol. Ann.* 6:337–363, 1971.

2

Immunological Findings in Hodgkin's and Non-Hodgkin's Lymphomas

James A. Goeken, M.D., Kathy Foucar, M.D.

Introduction

Traditional classifications of the malignant lymphomas have relied upon histopathology and correlation with clinical behavior. Recent progress in immunological studies has led to the understanding of normal lymphoid functions, to the recognition of specific functional lymphocyte subpopulations, and to the description of stages of lymphocyte maturation and development. These immunological findings can be readily applied to malignant lymphomas. We recognize three types of lymphocytes: B lymphocytes, which produce immunoglobulin molecules and hence are related to the humoral immune system; T lymphocytes, which are the effector cells of the cellular immune system; and non-T, non-B (null) lymphocytes, which are a heterogeneous group of cells that lack both standard T and B cell markers. Malignant lymphomas can arise from all stages of lymphocyte maturation and exhibit B-cell, T-cell or null-cell features. It is now possible to routinely analyze tissue, blood, and other body fluids for B, T and null cells and combine these studies with standard morphological evaluation to distinguish neoplastic from non-neoplastic lymphoid disorders. Immunological studies can identify the cell origin and define the stage of maturation at which the malignant cells are arrested. New functional classifications of non-Hodgkin's lymphomas have been based upon the use of these immunological lymphocyte studies. Specific immunological characteristics of cells have proven to be useful in predicting prognosis and in determining therapeutic measures in both the non-Hodgkin's lymphomas and related disorders such as lymphocytic leukemias.

In Hodgkin's disease, controversy still prevails concerning the etiology of the malignant cell, and no immunological classification has as yet been proposed. Immunological studies at present do not define Hodgkin's disease although they may support that diagnosis by excluding the diagnosis of non-Hodgkin's lymphoma. Immunological studies are also useful in the continuing search for the origin of the malignant cell of Hodgkin's disease and may well help us in understanding the pathophysiology of this entity.

This chapter will review the basic techniques used in the immunological evaluation of lymphoproliferative diseases and review the characteristic findings in the non-Hodgkin's lymphomas, Hodgkin's disease, and benign non-neoplastic disorders frequently called pseudolymphomas.

Cells of the Immune System

B Lymphocytes

B lymphocytes arise from bone marrow stem cells and are characterized by immunoglobulin (Ig) synthesis. In response to foreign antigens, normal B cells are stimulated to produce Ig and this functions in protecting the body against most bacterial, some viral, and possibly protozoal infections. The immunoglobulins (Ig) are a heterogeneous group of molecules, each of which consists of at least one basic unit or monomer, which is composed of four polypeptide chains. One pair of identical polypeptide chains called heavy (H) chains is joined with another identical pair of polypeptide chains of lower molecular weight called light (L) chains to form an Ig that can be represented by the general formula H_2L_2. There are five classes of H chains designated alpha (α), gamma (γ), mu (μ), delta (δ) and epsilon (ϵ), and two types of L-chains, kappa (κ) and lambda (λ). Any single B lymphocyte produces only one type of L-chain during its lifetime, although these cells may during the course of their maturation sequentially produce more than one type of H-chain of immunoglobulin. All progeny of a given B lymphocyte produce the same type of immunoglobulin L-chain and are said to constitute a clone. A monoclonal proliferation of B lymphocytes thus includes all cells derived from a single parent cell. Clinically evident monoclonal proliferation of lymphocytes are neoplastic processes, while those proliferations composed of multiple clones (polyclonal) are non-neoplastic processes. These B cells can be identified by demonstrating the presence of either surface or cytoplasmic immunoglobulin. Some B lymphocytes possess receptors for the third component of complement (C_3), for the Fc end of Ig (which functions to bind to antigen-antibody complexes) and for Epstein-Barr viruses. Certain B lymphocyte-specific membrane antigens have been identified and have begun to find application in the immunological identification of lymphocytes. Pre-B lymphocytes are immature B cells that have cytoplasmic μ heavy chain but have not yet begun to synthesize light chain. They lack surface immunoglobulin.

Plasma Cells

B lymphocytes may mature into plasma cells that produce and secrete large amounts of Ig. Plasma cells have abundant basophilic cytoplasm and an eccentric nucleus with chromatin characteristically clumped in a radial "clock-face" pattern. They usually possess generous quantities of cytoplasmic Ig (CIg) but little or no surface Ig (SIg). Plasma cells are terminally differentiated B lymphocytes.

T Lymphocytes

T lymphocytes are the effector cells of cell-mediated immunity and function in skin test delayed hypersensitivity reactions, transplant rejection, and protection from viruses, fungi, and intracellular bacteria, notably *Mycobacteria*. Immunoregulation is the function of certain subsets of T lymphocytes called helper and suppressor cells. Helper T cells stimulate B lymphocytes to mature into Ig-producing plasma cells while suppressor T cells inhibit Ig production by B cells and decrease the responsiveness of cytotoxic/effector T lymphocytes.

T lymphocytes are identified by their ability to spontaneously bind sheep red blood cells (s-rbc) to form rosettes (s-ER). Mature T cells form s-ER only at 4°C, while immature T cells (thymocytes) form s-ER at 37°C. T lymphocytes possess specific cell membrane antigens and a variety of these antigens have now been identified and found to have either general distribution on T cells or to be limited to a specific subset—for example, helper or suppressor T lymphocytes. Precursors of T lymphocytes, termed pre-T cells, possess T lymphocyte antigens but lack the ability to form s-ER. A monoclonal T cell proliferation is considered to be neoplastic whereas a polyclonal proliferation is benign, as was true for B lymphocytes.

Null Lymphocytes

Null lymphocytes lack standard immunological markers for B and T lymphocytes, but morphologically resemble lymphocytes, lymphoblasts, or transformed lymphocytes. These cells have also been referred to as non-T, non-B lymphocytes. This group probably contains several subpopulations, including precursors of B and T lymphocytes, K lymphocytes (the effector cells of the antibody-dependent cell cytotoxicity system) and the natural killer (NK) lymphocytes which are felt to play a role in tumor immunity.

Care must be taken in reading the literature for information about "null" cells since different authors have used different definitions for these cells. Some have used this term, as is used in this chapter, to include any lymphoid cell lacking SIg or ER functions regardless of other differentiation markers while others have used the "null" category exclusively for cells devoid of any detectable lymphocyte membrane antigens or receptors.

Macrophages (Histiocytes)

Macrophages, histiocytes, and monocytes are bone marrow-derived phagocytic cells with a common origin. They have been shown in many instances to be interconvertible; those in the peripheral blood are called monocytes while those present in tissues are macrophages or histiocytes. These cells interact with lymphocytes but are distinct from them and are involved in immunoregulation as well as phagocytosis. Macrophages possess receptors for immunoglobulin and complement, which function to facilitate both phagocytosis of antibody and/or complement-coated cells or foreign materials and also the presentation of antigens to lymphocytes.

Organ Localization of Normal Lymphocyte Populations

The normal adult peripheral blood lymphocyte population consists of approximately 60% to 80% T lymphocytes, 5% to 15% B lymphocytes, and 10% to 20% non-T, non-B lymphocytes. T lymphocytes circulate freely between blood and tissues. They are derived from bone marrow stem cells which are processed through the thymus and undergo differentiation there before entering the circulation again.

The T lymphocytes preferentially localize in the paracortical areas of the lymph nodes and the periarteriolar sheath of the spleen. Certain T lymphocytes also have a propensity to home to the dermis. B lymphocytes originate from bone marrow stem cells, and following maturation in the bone marrow, the site of B cell development, home to the follicles and medullary cords of the lymph nodes, follicles of the spleen, and to Peyer's patches in the gut wall. Macrophages are found within the sinuses of the lymph nodes and within the red pulp of the spleen, but they are also found in small numbers in all other immunologic regions of the spleen and lymph nodes. They comprise approximately 10% of peripheral blood white cells. A diagram of normal lymph node architecture showing location of T and B lymphocyte areas is shown in Figure 1.

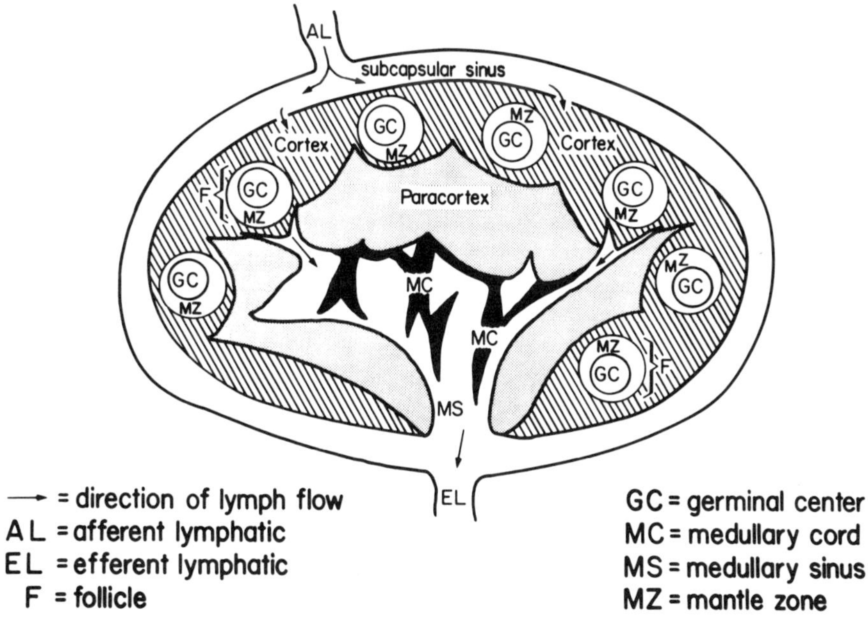

Figure 1: A diagram of normal lymph node architecture demonstrates the structural relationships of B lymphoid areas (cortex and medullary cords) and T lymphoid area (paracortex). The germinal centers and surrounding mantle zones are areas of B lymphocyte proliferation in response to antigenic stimulation. Maturing B lymphocytes and the immunoglobulin-secreting plasma cells come to rest in the medullary cords. Lymphocyte movement through the lymph node follows the direction of lymph flow (→), entering the subcapsular sinus via different lymphatic vessels (AL), and percolating through the cortex and paracortex toward the medullary sinus and eventually exiting via the efferent lymphatic vessels (EL).

Immunological Techniques for Lymphocyte and Macrophage Identification

Four different categories of cell markers are used to identify lymphocytes and macrophages: (1) secreted surface markers such as immunoglobulin, (2) cell membrane differentiation antigens, (3) cell enzymes, and (4) cell membrane receptors. Labeled antibody techniques such as immunofluorescence and immunoperoxidase staining are frequently used to identify surface membrane (or cytoplasmic) immunoglobulin, differentiation antigens, and certain enzymes. Cell surface receptors are commonly detected by rosetting techniques employing coated or uncoated erythrocytes or other types of particles including latex and zymosan.

These immunological techniques for identification of lymphocytes and macrophages may be performed on a variety of types of tissues. Certain of these assays require use of fresh tissue from which viable cells are extracted and suspended in a fluid medium, i.e., cell suspensions. Both immunofluorescence and immunoperoxidase staining techniques may be performed on frozen sections using monospecific antisera to detect surface membrane or cytoplasmic antigens. Routinely fixed paraffin-embedded material may be used to detect cytoplasmic immunoglobulin or lysozyme by the immunoperoxidase technique, but this technique is not satisfactory for detecting surface immunoglobulin or many cell membrane differentiation antigens.

Both the cell suspension and the tissue section methods have advantages and disadvantages. Suspension studies allow quantitative analysis of the cells that are present in a specimen taken from peripheral blood, bone marrow, lymph node, or tumor. An inherent difficulty with the use of the suspension techniques is the potential for selective loss of certain types of cells in the preparation of the suspension. Another problem involves the potential death of cells during the preparation of the suspension. Both problems lead to errors in quantitation, if not complete misinterpretation. Tissue section immunological preparations have the advantage of simultaneous morphological and immunological correlation. This is often quite helpful, particularly when evaluating a neoplasm that partially involves an organ or lymph node. Sections have the advantage of convenience in processing since they may be stained at any time because the cells do not need to be living in order to detect the antigens of interest. Sections have the disadvantages of difficulties in quantitating the cells present and in detecting certain membrane antigens that are present in small quantities. The latter problem is often due partially to "nonspecific" or background staining, which is encountered in immunofluorescence and immunoperoxidase staining techniques. Another disadvantage to sectioned material is that certain antigens are very labile and are destroyed by either fixation or freezing. Ideally, both the cell suspension and tissue section immunological studies should be performed on lymphomas for the most complete and comprehensive evaluation possible.

Identification of T and B Lymphocytes and Monocytes/Macrophages

A variety of immunological techniques are available for identifying T and B lymphocytes and monocytes (macrophages, histiocytes). The commonly used techniques are listed in Table 1.

Surface Immunoglobulin

The chief characteristic of B lymphocytes is their ability to synthesize immunoglobulin. Immunoglobulin is manufactured by the lymphocyte within the cytoplasm and then transferred to the cell membrane. The earliest identifiable B lymphocytes contain small quantities of the μ heavy chain without corresponding L-chain within their cytoplasm (so-called pre-B cells). With further differentiation,

Table 1
Immunological Markers of Lymphocytes and Monocytes

	Unique Properties	*Shared Properties*
B lymphocytes	Surface immunoglobulin (SIg)	C_3 receptors
	Cytoplasmic immunoglobulin (CIg)±	Fc receptors (±)
	E rosette–mouse (±)	Ia
	B cell surface antigens	
T lymphocytes	E rosette–sheep	C_3 receptors (±)
	T cell surface antigens	Fc receptors (±)
		Ia (±)
Null lymphocytes		Fc receptors (±)
		Ia
Monocytes*	Phagocytosis	C_3 receptors
	Adhere to glass	Fc receptors
	Lysozyme (muramidase)	Ia

*Similar markers are also present on macrophages and histiocytes
±May or may not be present

B lymphocytes begin to move IgM and IgD on to their cell membranes (Fig. 2). At this stage of development, cytoplasmic immunoglobulin is not detectable. With antigenic stimulation, B lymphocytes may switch from a primary immune response-associated immunoglobulin (IgM) to a secondary immune response-related immunoglobulin (IgG, IgA or IgE). With further maturation these cells lose their surface immunoglobulin and develop large amounts of easily detectable cytoplasmic immunoglobulin as they differentiate into plasma cells. In most cases, except for the early unstimulated small lymphocyte, which simultaneously possesses both surface membrane IgM and IgD, the B lymphocytes bear one heavy chain and one light chain of immunoglobulin at a time.

Leukemias and lymphomas of B cell origin that possess detectable surface or cytoplasmic immunoglobulin bear a single type of light chain and either one or two heavy chains. Such malignancies are

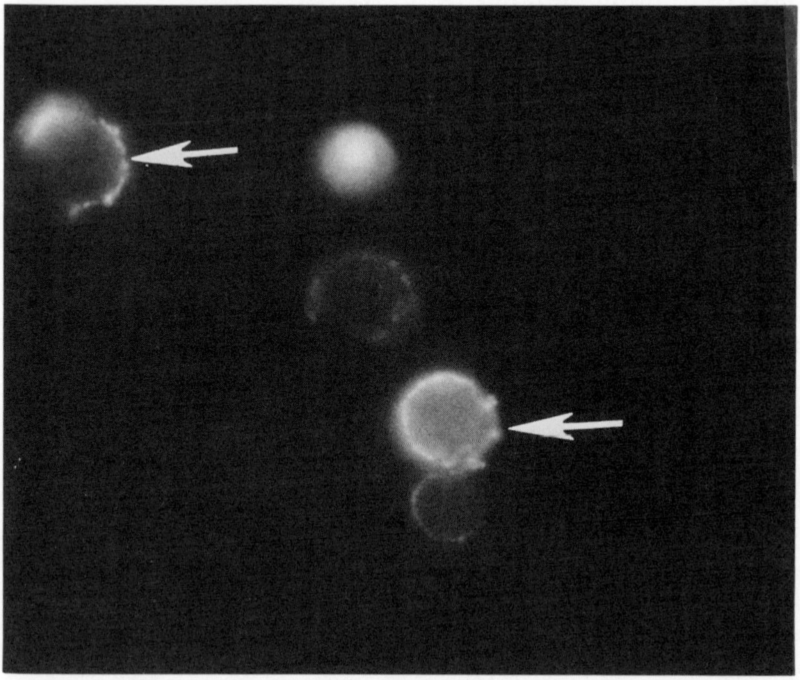

Figure 2: Immunofluorescence photomicrograph of a cell suspension containing B lymphocytes stained for μ-heavy chain of IgM. Cell surface membranes are outlined (→) by the fluoresceinated antibody. (Magnification = ×1200)

referred to as monoclonal. In contrast, a non-neoplastic lymphoid population contains cells that bear a spectrum of heavy and light chain types of immunoglobulin and are referred to as polyclonal proliferations. The presence of a monoclonal pattern of surface or cytoplasmic immunoglobulin is very convincing evidence of a B cell malignancy, whereas the presence of polyclonal staining for immunoglobulin in a lymphoid population is presumptive evidence of a benign process.

B and T Lymphocyte Surface Antigens

B lymphocyte cell membranes possess certain antigens that can be identified with antisera or monoclonal antibodies. In several cases, these antigens are shared with granulocytes and/or monocytes. They are useful in identifying B cell-derived neoplasms that are either insufficiently well differentiated to make immunoglobulins or are nonsecretory due to a defective synthetic apparatus. Table 2 contains a list of some of these reagents which can be obtained from commercial sources.

Monoclonal antibodies or antisera can be used to detect a number of T lymphocyte-specific cell membrane antigens. Certain of the differentiation antigens are common to all but the earliest stages of T cell maturation and development, while others are specific for functional subclasses of T lymphocytes, for example, the helper and suppressor cells. Hybridoma-produced anti-T cell antibodies have become available from commercial sources and promise to be a significant addition to the immunopathologist's diagnostic armamentarium. A list of some available products and their specificities is given in Table 3.

Immune recognition and response in man is controlled by genetic material localized to chromosome 6 and called the major histocompatibility complex (MHC). A component of the MHC in the mouse (in which the structure is more fully understood than it is in man) is the Ia region whose gene products are involved with self-recognition. The analogue in man is the DR locus which produces Ia-like gene products that are expressed by many types of human cells including B lymphocytes, some T lymphocyte subsets, macrophages, epidermal cells, and sperm cells. Table 2 contains a list of some anti-Ia reagents available. They have been employed in diagnostic immunopathology to identify undifferentiated neoplasm of lymphoreticular origin. B cell and true histiocytic neoplasms are typically Ia-positive (+) while undifferentiated carcinomas, T cell lymphomas, and nonhematopoietic sarcomas are usually Ia-negative (−).

Table 2
Monoclonal Antibodies with B Lymphocyte or Other Specificities

Specificity	*Antibody(ies)*	*Commercial Source(s)*	*Comments*
Pan-B cell	B-1	Coulter	Reacts with all B lymphocytes except plasma cells. Does not react with T cells, granulocytes, or monocytes.
	BA-1	Hybritech	Detects an antigen present on all B cells, B cell lymphomas, monocytes, and granulocytes. Occasionally ⊕ in malignant melanoma and neuroblastoma. Negative on T cells and on plasma cells.
	BA-2	Hybritech	Reacts with a subset of B cells, some T-ALL cases, some CLL, AML, and AMML cases as well as a few epithelial malignancies, neuroblastoma, and some melanomas.
Anti-Ia(DR)	OKI-1	Ortho	
	anti-HLA-DR	Becton-Dickinson	
	I-2	Coulter	
	anti-Ia	New England Nuclear	
Common ALL antigen	J-5	Coulter	Reacts with immature B and T lymphocytes. Positive in 70% of ALL cases and 35% of nodular NHL.
	BA-3	Hybritech	
NK, K cells	Leu-7	Becton-Dickinson	

Table 3
Monoclonal Antibodies with T Lymphocyte Specificities

Specificity	*Antibody(ies)*	*Commercial Source(s)*	*Comments*
Pan-T cell	Leu-1	Becton-Dickinson	These react with all stages of T cells. Some (Leu-1, Lyt-2, T 101) also react with CLL/WDLL B cells.
	OKT-1	Ortho	
	T-101	Hybritech	
	Lyt-2	New England Nuclear	
Mature T cell	Leu-4	Becton-Dickinson	React with postthymic "peripheral T cells" only
	OKT-3	Ortho	
s-ER ⊕ T cells	Leu-5	Becton-Dickinson	Specific for the sheep rbc receptor.
	OKT-11	Ortho	
	Lyt-3	New England Nuclear	
	T-11	Coulter	
Helper/inducer T cells	Leu-3a	Becton-Dickinson	
	T-4	Coulter	
	OKT-4	Ortho	
	Lyt-1	New England Nuclear	
Cytotoxic/suppressor T cells	OKT-8	Ortho	
	T-8a	Coulter	
	Leu-2a	Becton-Dickinson	
Thymocytes	OKT-6	Ortho	
	Leu-6	Becton-Dickinson	
Early thymocytes	OKT-9	Ortho	

Cell Membrane Receptors

Rosette techniques are used to detect complement receptors, sheep erythrocyte receptors, and Fc receptors.

Complement Receptors (CR)

Most B cells, except the plasma cell, bear a receptor for the third component of complement (C_3). Complement receptors are identified by means of a rosetting technique employing erythrocytes that have been sensitized with IgM antibody and then reacted with a source of complement. This sensitized cell will bind to any lymphocyte possessing a receptor for C_3. The rosette that forms is termed an EAC rosette (Erythrocyte Antibody Complement) (Fig. 3). Complement receptors are not specific for B lymphocytes because at certain early stages of differentiation T lymphocytes also possess them. In addition, certain nonlymphoid cells, including macrophages, granulocytes, and some tissue cells possess complement receptors. Nevertheless, the complement receptor is often a very useful marker for the B lymphocyte, particularly in peripheral blood and lymph nodes. Complement receptors are generally detected in suspension studies, although they may be performed on frozen sections of lymph node or other tissue.

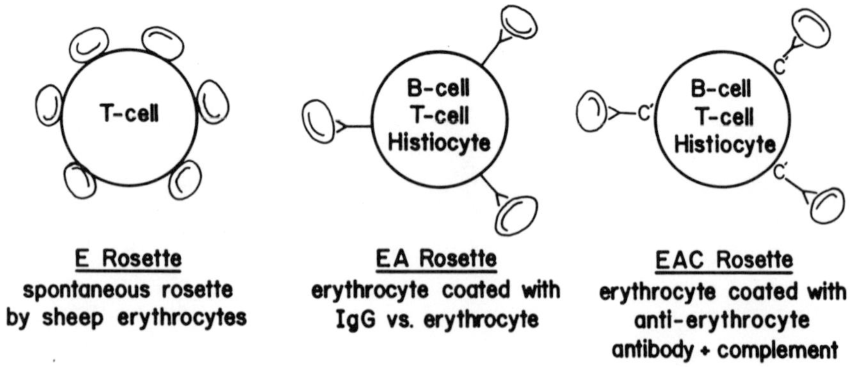

Figure 3: Schematic drawing of spontaneous rosette formation with sheep erythrocytes (left), erythrocytes coated with antibody (center), and erythrocytes coated with antibody and complement (right). Cells likely to demonstrate these rosette properties are indicated.

Erythrocyte Receptors

T lymphocytes are characterized by their ability to form spontaneous rosettes with sheep erythrocytes (s-ER) (Fig. 3). S-ER studies are usually performed in cell suspensions where the percentage of rosetting cells can be determined. Clinical studies of suspected T cell malignancies require that the s-ER positive cells be stained and microscopically examined to determine if the rosetting cells are cytologically malignant or benign. A few investigators have reported success in performing ER studies on frozen sections, but this has been difficult for many laboratories to reproduce. With the availability of T lymphocyte-specific monoclonal antibodies, it appears unnecessary to pursue tissue section ER techniques.

Fc Receptors

The Fc receptor (FcR) binds the Fc end of the immunoglobulin molecule which is its "constant" region where immunoglobulin class specificity determinants reside, as contrasted with the Fab or antibody-binding end of the molecule. FcRs are not specific for any type of lymphocyte, being present on some T cells and null cells, certain tissue cells, most B cells, as well as monocyte/macrophages, and granulocytes. For this reason, FcRs are of *limited value* in identifying cells. It is of interest to note that T lymphocytes that bear FcRs appear to be of two types. Those with IgM-FcR appear to function as helper cells while IgG-FcR ⊕ cells demonstrate suppressor activity.

The Fcγ receptor (IgG-FcR) is detected with sheep erythrocytes coated with antisheep erythrocyte antibodies of IgG type (Fig. 3). Such IgG-coated erythrocytes rosette with cells possessing Fc receptors, forming EA-rosettes. Fc receptors are also detectable with heat-aggregated IgG tagged with fluorescein. Fcμ receptors specific for IgM (IgM-FcR) are detected in a similar fashion using IgM, rather than IgG, to coat sheep erythrocytes.

Enzymes

Terminal Deoxynucleotidyl Transferase (TdT)

This enzyme is a unique DNA polymerase that adds deoxynucleotides to the 3′ hydroxyl end of single-stranded poly- or oligodeoxynucleotides without template direction. It has proved to be a useful marker for both T and null lymphoblasts in acute lymphoblastic leukemia and lymphoblastic lymphomas as well as for the lymphoid-type blast cells that develop in the blast crisis of chronic granulocytic leukemias. Normal bone marrow contains less than 2% TdT ⊕ blast cells. Thymocytes contain TdT, but other lymphoid tissues and peripheral blood do not contain TdT ⊕ cells.

This enzyme was originally measured biochemically, but commercially available antisera have proved to be a very sensitive means of identifying TdT ⊕ cells using immunofluorescence or immunoperoxidase microscopic techniques. Air-dried touch imprints of tissue, blood smears, and frozen tissue sections can all be used for evaluation for presence of TdT (Fig. 4).

Application of Lymphocyte Marker Studies to Disease Diagnosis

Reactive or Hyperplastic Lymph Nodes

Many reactive processes within lymph nodes are morphologically difficult to distinguish from malignant lymphoma. Surface marker analysis can facilitate morphological diagnosis of equivocal biopsies by establishing the monoclonal or polyclonal nature of the process. For example, in follicular hyperplasia, the germinal centers are numerous and can mimic a nodular lymphoma. However, the reactive germinal centers contain polyclonal B lymphocytes which can be documented on frozen sections by immunofluorescence techniques or in formalin-fixed, paraffin-embedded sections by immunoperoxidase methods (Fig. 5). Characteristically, germinal centers will contain both κ and λ light chain-positive cells in ratios approximating 2:1 which is the normal for B lymphocytes in peripheral blood. Multiple heavy chains are often demonstrated in these reactive processes as well, although the percentages are variable depending on the duration of the antigenic stimulus and the individual patient involved. Sometimes atypical reactive processes result in effacement of lymph node architecture and obliteration of germinal centers. In these cases, immunofluorescence or immunoperoxidase methods can also be employed to verify that the proliferating cells are polyclonal. Hyperplastic histiocytes within sinuses can be identified by immunoperoxidase staining for lysozyme (muramidase).

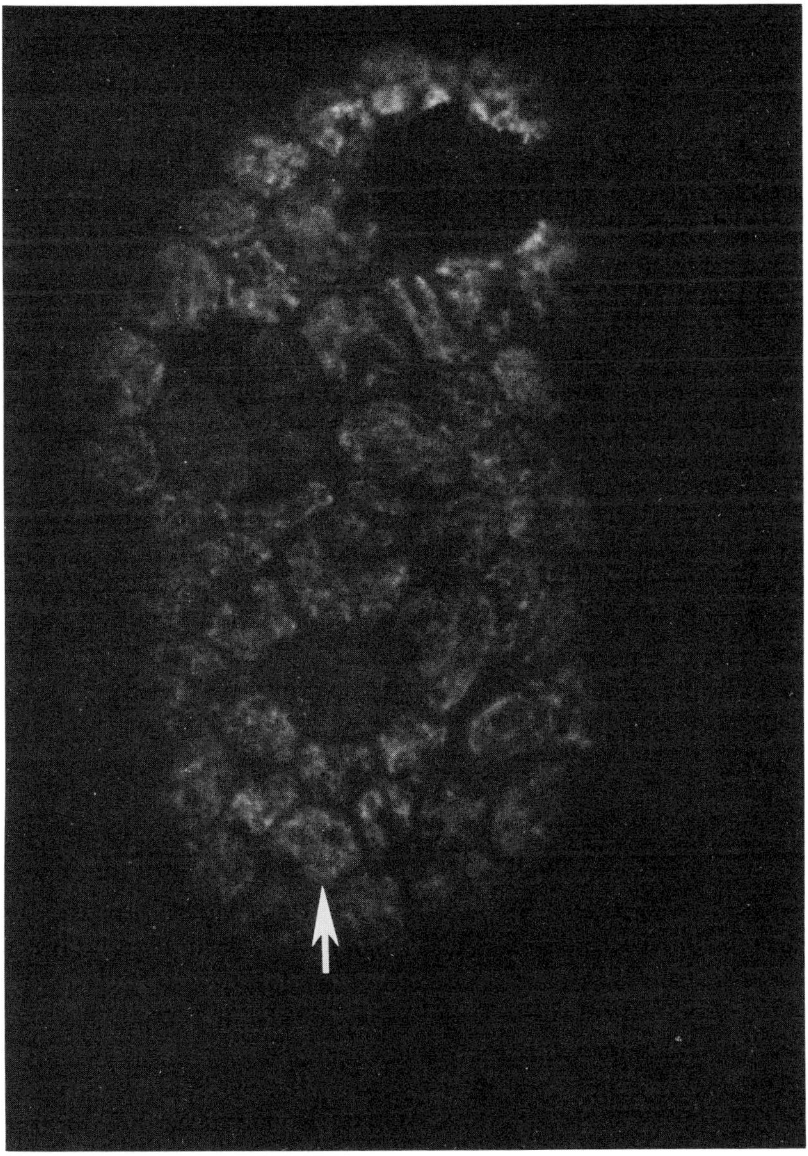

Figure 4: Immunofluorescence staining of an air-dried cytocentrifuged preparation of acute lymphoblastic leukemia cells for terminal deoxynucleotidyl transferase (TdT) showing the characteristic stippled intranuclear staining (→). (Magnification = ×1200)

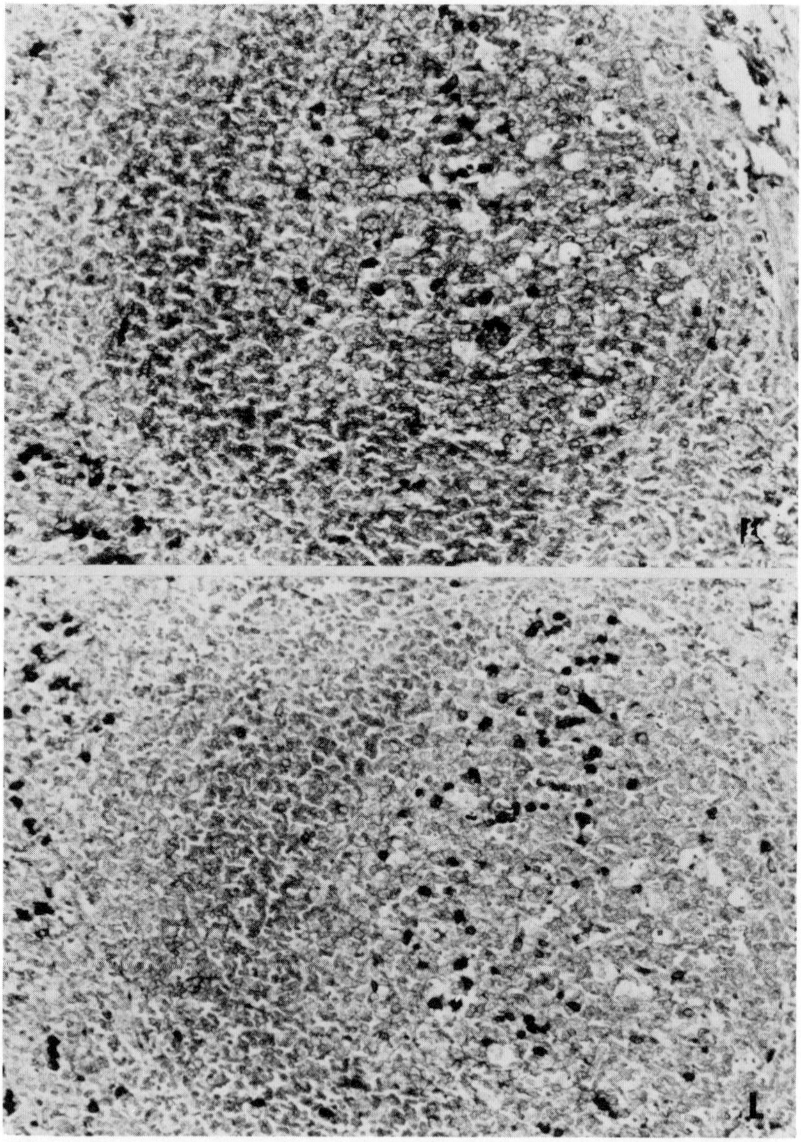

Figure 5: A normal lymphoid follicle contains B lymphocytes of both kappa and lambda type. The normal ratio is two kappa: one lambda producing cell. The variable staining intensity of the cells is also characteristic of normal follicles. In this composite photomicrograph, the same follicle has been stained by the immunoperoxidase technique for kappa (K) and (L) light chains. (Magnification = ×135)

Pseudolymphomas

Extranodal reactive lymphoid hyperplasias are often referred to as pseudolymphomas because they may form bulky tumors, invade and disrupt normal anatomy, and have a histological resemblance to malignant non-Hodgkin's lymphomas. The occurrence and histological features have been reviewed in Chapter 1. Morphological evaluation of invasive lymphoid infiltrates in practically any organ may be inadequate to separate benign from malignant processes so that immunological studies are increasingly widely employed to establish the correct diagnosis. Pseudolymphomas and nodal reactive lymphoid hyperplasias are indistinguishable on immunological grounds in that each is comprised of polyclonal B lymphocytes, mature T cells, and plasma cells (Table 4). A normal mantle zone of SIgM and SIgD ⊕ cells surrounds the follicles and separates them from the T cell zone beyond. In contrast to the nodular and diffuse B cell lymphomas, SIg density varies considerably from cell to cell in pseudolymphomas and reactive lymphoid hyperplasias. Cell suspension studies on benign reactive processes demonstrate that considerable variation exists from case to case in quantitative lymphocyte surface marker results. Most commonly, the percentage of B lymphocytes is increased and T lymphocytes decreased when compared with normal lymph node populations. When monospecific antisera are used to enumerate heavy and light chains on B cells, one finds increases in all classes of heavy chains and both types of light chains.

In some cases, there may be a blurring of the distinction between benign pseudolymphomas and malignant lymphomas. Reports of persistent reactive lymphoid hyperplasias progressively evolving into large cell variants of lymphoma (diffuse histiocytic or immunoblastic lymphoma) can be found in the literature, although this is an unusual event. Many of the patients in whom this malignant transformation

Table 4
Immunological Markers in Normal Lymph Nodes, Reactive Hyperplasia, and Pseudolymphoma*

Tissue	*N=*	*Diagnosis*	*s-ER +*	*SIg +*
Lymph node	16	Normal	68 (61–77)	18 (12–28)
Lymph node	85	Reactive hyperplasia	46 (18–59)	35 (12–50)
Various	15	Pseudolymphoma	60 (31–68)	41 (11–62)

*Data assembled from multiple reports in the literature
+ Mean and range

has occurred have had underlying immunoregulatory disorders, such as connective tissue or immunodeficiency diseases, or have been iatrogenically immunosuppressed for purposes of organ transplantation. In most reports, the malignant transformation is accompanied by the replacement of the polyclonal population with a monoclonal one, usually of B lymphocyte type. Scattered cases of an apparently polyclonal lymphoid expansion in a neoplastic fashion, eventually causing the death of the patient, have been reported generally in the context of posttransplantation immunosuppression. Such examples may represent viral-induced lymphocyte transformation and proliferation which is uncontrollable in the face of depressed or absent T cell immunoregulatory function. Epstein-Barr virus infection has been associated with such events.

In most patients, reactive lymphoid hyperplasias and pseudolymphomas remain benign. If they persist and behave aggressively in patients with such diseases as systemic lupus erythematosus or Sjögren's syndrome or in the postrenal transplant patient, immunological reevaluation should be considered despite previous reports of a benign polyclonal process, since malignant transformations are up to 100 times more common in these individuals than in the normal population.

Non-Hodgkin's Lymphomas

The non-Hodgkin's lymphomas (NHL) represent a clinically and morphologically heterogeneous group of diseases arising from lymphocytes in various stages of maturation or transformation. Only a rare case of NHL arises from true histiocytes or macrophages. It is thought that the lymphoma cells mimic, to a certain extent, their normal cell counterparts both morphologically and immunologically. As described in another chapter, certain morphological features (such as nodular growth pattern) almost always indicate the derivation of the neoplastic clone; however, cases of NHL are frequently difficult to subclassify using morphological criteria alone. Distinction from atypical benign processes can also be difficult. Because these problems of morphological interpretation are common, surface marker analysis is frequently helpful to substantiate morphological diagnosis. An immunological categorization of NHL reveals that 80% of cases of NHL are of B cell derivation, 15% are T cell, and 5% lack surface markers (null cell). True histiocytic lymphomas are rare and usually represent less than 1% of NHL. Specific criteria for establishing monoclonality of B cell neoplasms are somewhat arbitrary; however, some guidelines for interpreting lymphocyte surface marker results can be suggested. It is necessary to examine not only the absolute number of B cells present but also the ratio of cells bearing different heavy chains and light chains of immunoglobulin to distinguish between benign and malignant conditions. One author suggests that a monoclonal B cell population is present if (1) the κ to λ ratio is ≥3:1, or (2) the λ to κ ratio is ≥2:1, and (3) one heavy chain predominates over the sum of the other three by ≥3:1 (except in the cases of IgM and IgD which may be present simultaneously on certain neoplastic cells). Table 5 shows both the traditional classification system for NHL devised by Rappaport and the immunological classification of cases of NHL by morphological subtype derived from multiple series of cases. It must be noted that the term "histiocytic" in the Rappaport classification is used to describe large mononuclear cells, although these large cells have now been found in the vast majority of cases to be transformed lymphocytes.

Nodular Lymphomas

The presence of a definite nodular growth pattern establishes that an NHL is derived from follicular (germinal center) cells and is thus

Table 5
Immunological Classification of Non-Hodgkin's Lymphoma

Morphological Classification (Rappaport)	*Immunological Classification*
Well-differentiated lymphocytic lymphoma, diffuse	98–100% B cell, 2% T cell
Poorly differentiated lymphocytic lymphoma, nodular	almost all B cell
Poorly differentiated lymphocytic lymphoma, diffuse	55% B cell, 30% T cell, 15% null cell
Mixed lymphocytic and "histiocytic" lymphoma, nodular	almost all B cell
Mixed lymphocytic and "histiocytic" lymphoma, diffuse	53% B, 47% T*
"Histiocytic" lymphoma, nodular	almost all B cell
"Histiocytic" lymphoma, diffuse	50–70% B cell, 5–30% T cell, 5–30% null cell
Burkitt's lymphoma	almost all B cell
Lymphoblastic lymphoma	predominantly T cell, few null cell

*Of 17 cases with immunological evaluation reported in the literature

of B cell origin. Immunofluorescence and immunoperoxidase studies have demonstrated monoclonal immunoglobulin in the nodules of nodular lymphoma in most cases evaluated (Fig. 6), although occasional examples are SIg ⊖. Nodular lymphomas can be composed primarily of small cleaved cells (poorly differentiated lymphocytic lymphoma), large cells (histiocytic lymphoma), or a mixture of small and large cells (mixed lymphocytic and histiocytic lymphoma); these cell types reflect the morphological diversity of the benign germinal center. Regardless of cell size, the immunological findings are similar. Intensity of the immunofluorescence staining reaction on nodular lymphoma cells is often greater than that seen on peripheral blood B lymphocytes but is similar to that of normal follicular center lymphocytes. The most common class of immunoglobulin associated with these follicular center cells is IgM. IgD and IgG are found somewhat less frequently and IgA is fairly uncommon. Strong complement receptors are also usually present on the B cells of nodular lymphomas. Normal T lymphocytes are often present in substantial numbers among the neoplastic B cells but these are morphologically normal. For this reason, it is very important to combine morphological studies with cell suspension immunological studies to avoid erroneous interpretation of the results.

Diffuse Lymphomas

This group of neoplasms is much more heterogeneous than the nodular lymphomas and immunologically may be B, T, or null. They are subdivided in the Rappaport classification, as are the nodular lymphomas, according to the size and cytological features of the principal cells in the neoplasm.

Well-Differentiated Lymphocytic Lymphoma (WDLL). WDLL is immunologically and morphologically similar to chronic lymphocytic leukemia (CLL) and most cases are composed of small bland-appearing B lymphocytes exhibiting weak SIgM or SIgM and D. Occasionally the SIg reaction is too weak to detect by immunofluorescence microscopy, although more sensitive techniques such as autoradiography confirm its presence. Weak C_3 receptors are present on most but not all B cell type WDLL cells. Only 2% of WDLL is derived from T lymphocytes as defined by presence of s-ER and mature T cell antigens; however, the cells of 80–90% of all WDLL and CLL cases react with certain pan-T monoclonal antibodies (T 101, Leu 1, and Lyt 2) including SIg ⊕ examples. Other B lymphoid neoplasms have not been observed to bear this or any other T cell antigens.

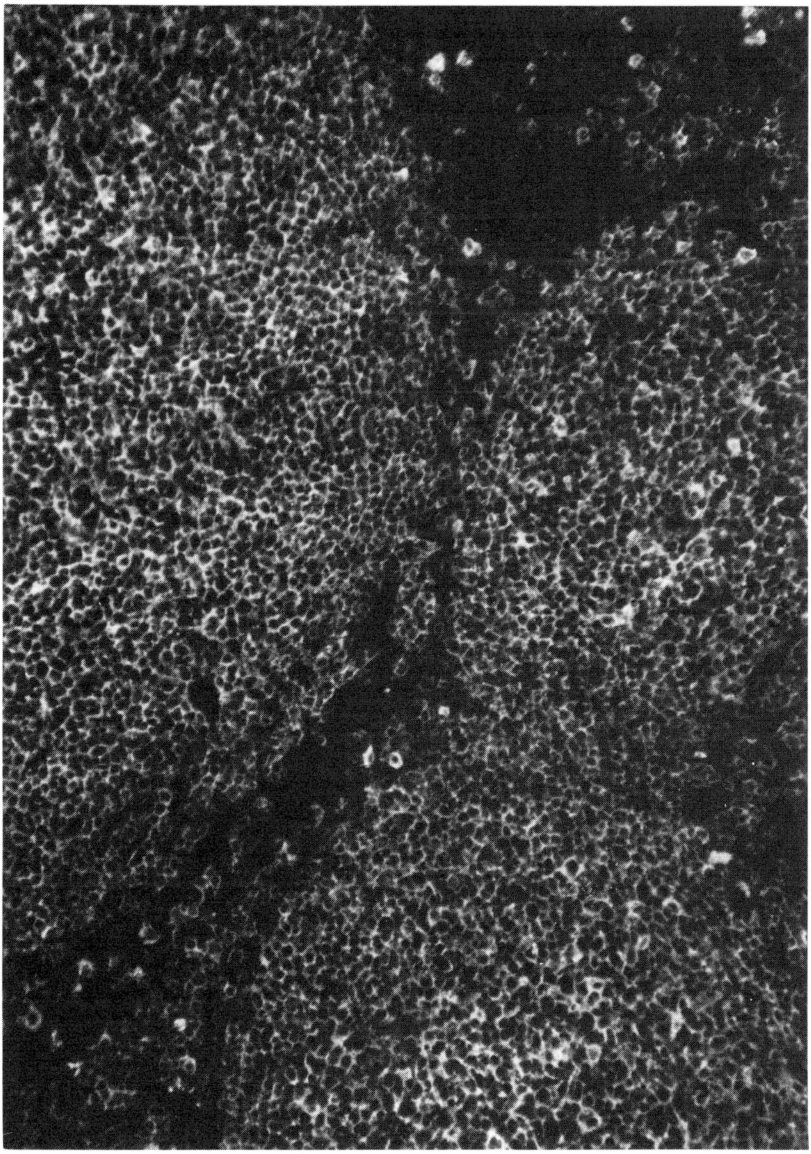

Figure 6: Nodular non-Hodgkin's lymphoma frozen tissue sections stained for μ-heavy chain (IgM). Three nodular growth centers of this lymphoma appear near confluence. Areas between nodules contain predominantly normal residual T and B lymphocytes, however, some lymphoma cells are also present. (Magnification = ×192)

Intermediately Differentiated Lymphocytic Lymphoma (IDLL). IDLL is a recently described type of NHL (and is not a specific category within the Rappaport classification) which apparently arises from a B lymphocyte of the mantle zone or lymphoid cuff of the germinal center. The immunological properties of these tumor cells are intermediate between those of WDLL and poorly differentiated lymphocytic lymphoma (PDLL). They are SIgM ⊕ and often are SIgD ⊕, as well. The density of SIg is greater than that of WDLL but less than PDLL. Complement receptors are usually present but are less avid than those of PDLL.

Poorly Differentiated Lymphocytic Lymphoma (PDLL). Although nodular PDLL is consistently of B lymphocyte origin, cases of diffuse PDLL may be derived from T cells, B cells, or null cells. About 55% of the cases have B lymphocyte markers. High density SIgM is the most frequently demonstrated surface immunoglobulin; less common are SIgG and SIgA. Striking uniformity of cell staining intensity is present in these tumors in contrast to the variable staining in a reactive B cell hyperplasia (Fig. 7). Complement receptors are usually present but are somewhat less avid than those associated with nodular PDLL.

T cell origin has been demonstrated for 15–30% of diffuse PDLL cases. These lymphomas are presumed to arise from postthymic or mature peripheral T lymphocytes. These cells selectively infiltrate the paracortex of lymph nodes and are cytologically very pleomorphic. Often these malignant cells are accompanied in the tumor by clusters of epithelioid histiocytes, eosinophils, and/or plasma cells, suggesting that these neoplastic T cells retain some immunological functions. Because of this marked morphological heterogeneity, immunological evaluation is helpful in establishing the diagnosis of T cell PDLL. The immunological markers of these cells include s-ER and IgM Fc receptors (Fig. 8). The cells of these lymphomas will react with one or more of the monoclonal antibodies to mature human T lymphocyte antigens, including the pan-T cell, mature T cell, helper/inducer T cell, and cytotoxic/suppressor T cell groups listed in Table 3. Several cases of this type have been proven to have the "helper" T cell phenotype which explains the presence of plasma cells and the accompanying polyclonal hypergammaglobulinemia. Production of migration inhibition factor, a lymphokine that immobilizes macrophages, could lead to the accumulations of histiocytes observed. Up to 15% of cases of diffuse PDLL are derived from null cells. Studies have indicated a worse prognosis for null cell lymphoma than the morphologically similar process possessing either T or B cell properties.

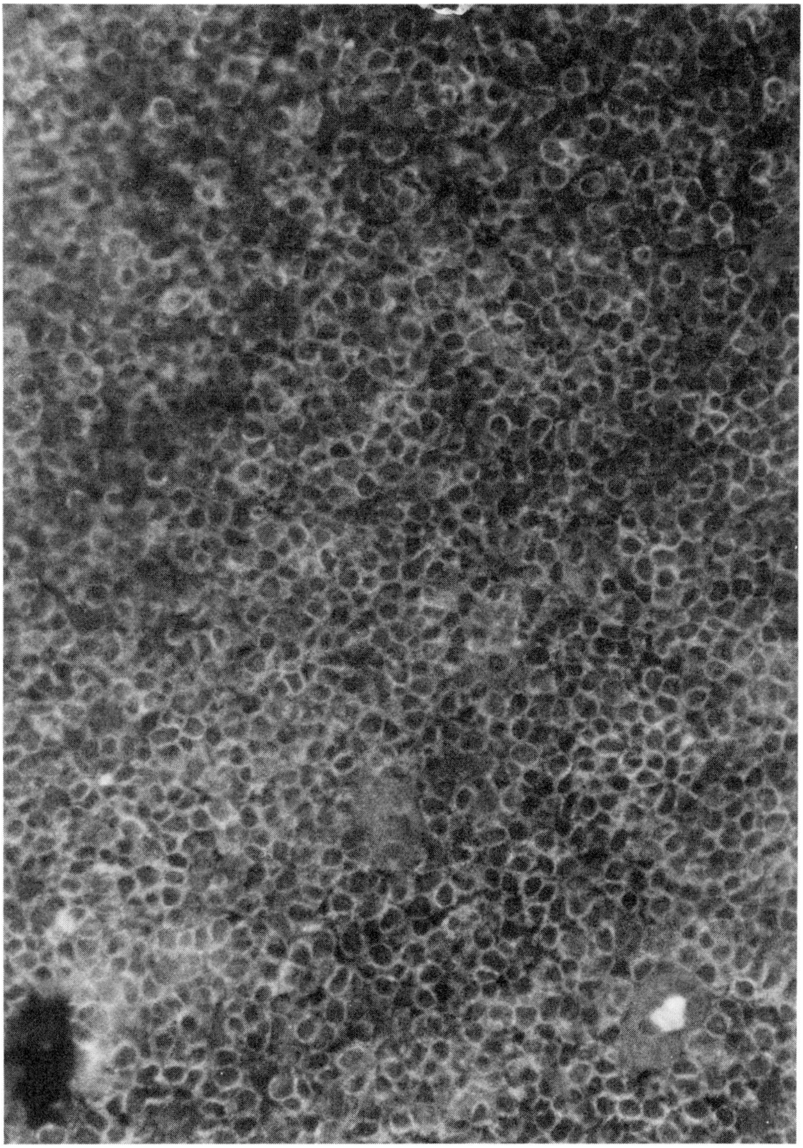

Figure 7: Diffuse non-Hodgkin's lymphoma (B cell) frozen tissue sections stained for α-heavy chain (IgA). Characteristic of such lymphomas is the extremely homogeneous staining, indicative of very uniform concentrations of immunoglobulin on the cell membranes. (Magnification = ×480)

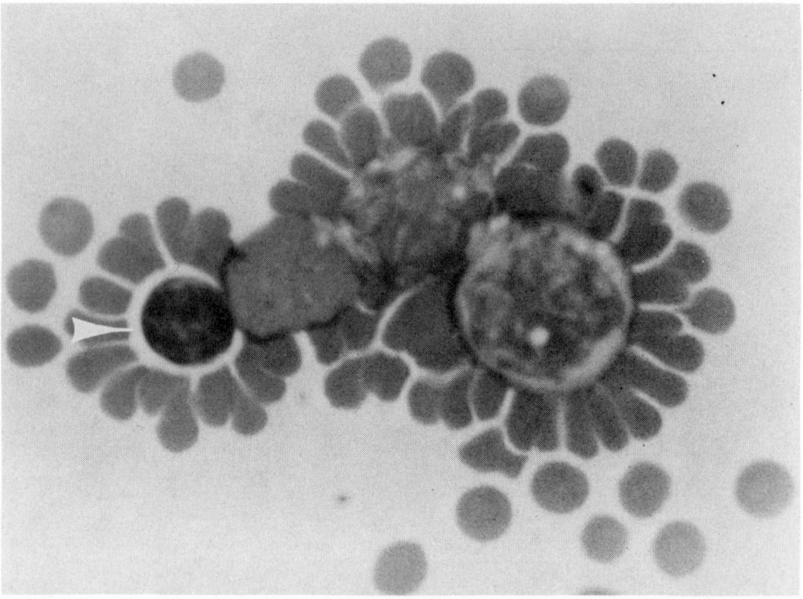

Figure 8: Cytocentrifuged s-ER preparations from a lymph node cell suspension from a case of T cell lymphoma. The larger cells rosetting with sheep erythrocytes are lymphoma cells while the smaller one (▷) is a normal mature T lymphocyte. (Magnification = ×1400)

Mixed Lymphocytic-Histiocytic and Histiocytic Lymphomas, Diffuse. Essentially, similar immunological findings are present in diffuse mixed and histiocytic (large cell) lymphomas as have been described in PDLL. About 60% of cases are of B lymphoid origin, 15–30% are T cell type, and 10–25% lack B or T markers. B cell mixed and large cell diffuse lymphomas are most often SIgM ⊕, although SIgG ⊕ cases are not unusual. Some examples have cytoplasmic Ig (Fig. 9). Complement receptors may or may not be present. Peripheral T cell lymphomas of large cell type have surface markers similar to those of diffuse T cell PDLL.

A subgroup of diffuse histiocytic lymphomas having the largest cells has been frequently referred to as immunoblastic lymphoma (IBL), immunoblastic sarcoma (IBS), or large cell, immunoblastic (Working Formulation). They are most often of B lymphoid origin, although T cell types have been reported. The B cell types may possess SIg or CIg or both. CR may be present in some cases. T cell types may be

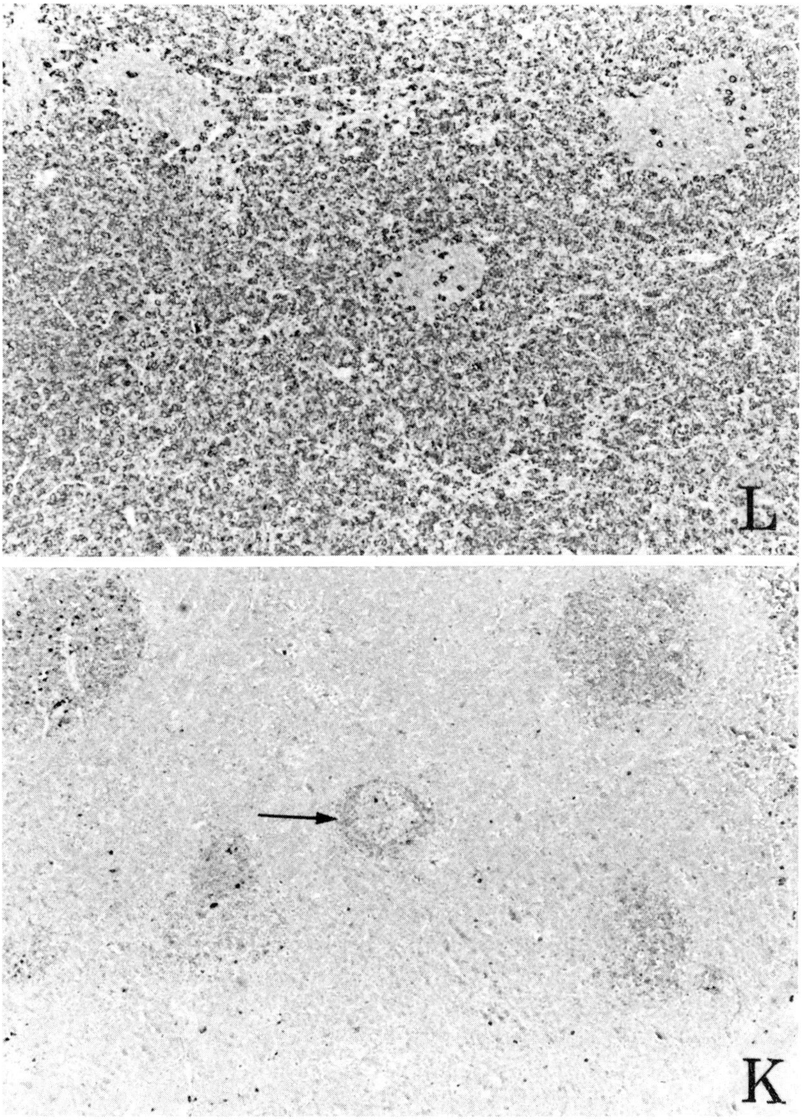

Figure 9: An example of diffuse mixed lymphoma, B cell type, demonstrating presence of cytoplasmic lambda light chain (L, darkly stained cells) and absence of kappa (K, nonstained). A few small foci of residual normal lymphocytes contain kappa positive cells (→). (Magnification = ×50)

s-ER ⊕/T lymphocyte antigen ⊕ or be T antigen ⊕ only. A number of cases have been of null cell type. It may be impossible to distinguish immunoblastic sarcoma from undifferentiated carcinoma on morphological grounds alone, and since some examples of IBL/IBS lack both SIg and s-ER, markers such as Ia, BA 1, or T 101 may be useful in making the diagnosis of lymphoma.

Rare cases of diffuse large cell lymphoma are derived from histiocytes and are thus true histiocytic lymphomas. They retain many morphological and immunological characteristics of benign histiocytes, such as complement and Fc receptors and abundant cytoplasmic lysozyme, which can be detected by immunoperoxidase staining. They lack monoclonal SIg, CIg, s-ER, and T lymphocyte surface antigens.

Lymphoblastic Lymphoma (LBL). Thymic T cell lymphomas were previously grouped with diffuse PDLL but have now been classified separately and termed lymphoblastic lymphomas. These tumors make up approximately 5% of the NHL and compose greater than 40% of all T cell lymphomas. They are characterized by lymphoblastic morphology often with distinctively convoluted nuclei.

Lymphoblastic lymphoma is commonly thought to be closely related to T cell acute lymphoblastic leukemia (T-ALL) and indeed there are many clinical, morphological, and immunological similarities between the two diseases. T-ALL presents primarily as a leukemic process with frequent secondary tissue infiltration, while in LBL tissue disease predominates. The mediastinum is frequently the site of disease in both LBL and T-ALL. These cell nuclei of both diseases are terminal deoxynucleotidyl transferase (TdT) positive (Fig. 4). As expected, most cases of lymphoblastic lymphoma are composed of T cells, although some cases lack surface markers. T-ALL and those cases of LBL derived from T cells are considered to be central T cell malignancies presumably arising from immature thymic lymphoid cells. Several subtypes have been identified corresponding to stages of differentiation of thymic T lymphocytes which can be identified by monoclonal antibodies (OKT 3, 6, 9).

Undifferentiated Lymphoma, Burkitt's, and Non-Burkitt's types. These tumors are uncommon types of NHL which are composed of intermediate sized cells that have been termed small, noncleaved cells in the Working Formulation. These cells, whether morphologically of the classical Burkitt type first described in African children or the more pleomorphic American Burkitt-like malignancy, have all been uniformly of B lymphocyte type when evaluated by surface marker studies. The cells possess SIgM in most cases, although SIgG is occasionally reported. Rarely, C_3 receptors or Fc receptors may be present.

Cutaneous T Cell Lymphomas. These include a number of morphologically and clinically related diseases, particularly mycosis fungoides, Sézary's syndrome, certain large cell diffuse lymphomas, and some well-differentiated lymphocytic lymphomas. Immunopathologic examination of the cutaneous T cell lymphomas has demonstrated that they are derived from helper T lymphocytes which form s-ER and possess surface membrane Fc receptors for IgM. They are OKT 3 ⊕/Leu 1 ⊕ and OKT 4 ⊕/Leu 3a ⊕. Many of the peripheral T cell lymphomas of helper phenotype demonstrate epidermal infiltration, which is an infrequent finding in cutaneous infiltrates of other types of lymphomas.

Lymphoplasmacytic Lymphomas. Although lymphoplasmacytic lymphoma is not a category in the Rappaport classification, this term is used in certain other lymphoma classifications. It refers to an uncommon type of lymphoma of diffuse pattern having a distinctive neoplastic cell population which includes a large number of plasmacytoid lymphocytes and plasma cells. These tumors arise from B cells of the medullary area of lymph nodes and they possess large quantities of cytoplasmic Ig, most commonly IgM with IgG and IgA seen in small numbers of cases. These cells often secrete monoclonal Ig, and patients may have a clinical picture similar to Waldenstrom's macroglobulinemia. These cells may possess SIg of the same class and type as is present in their cytoplasm. Complement receptors (CR) are absent.

Hodgkin's Disease

Hodgkin's disease is well established as a malignant clinicopathological entity, but the etiology of the malignant cells is still undefined. The histopathological classification in Hodgkin's disease, as defined by Lukes and Butler (see Chapter 1, *Pathology of Nodal and Extranodal Lymphoma*), recognizes four subtypes with strikingly different microscopic features.

The common features in all the subtypes are Reed-Sternberg (RS) cells and atypical large mononuclear cells (Hodgkin cells) which are set in a polymorphous background of cells including lymphocytes, macrophages, plasma cells, and eosinophils.

The proliferating malignant cell in Hodgkin's disease has been identified as the large mononuclear or "Hodgkin cell." Some authorities believe the Reed-Sternberg giant cell to be a nonproliferating cell, which is perhaps a polyploid product of an aberrant cell division.

Others have found DNA synthesis in RS cells. Hodgkin and RS cells constitute 10% of the tumor mass, an unusual situation in a malignancy, suggesting that the malignant cells may possess chemotactic activity which allow them to attract and surround themselves with the various types of inflammatory cells mentioned above. It is well recognized that patients with Hodgkin's disease have one or more immunological abnormalities accompanying their malignancy. Anergy due to defective cell-mediated immunity is common. This clinical evidence of a defect in T cell function has been confirmed and elaborated upon in a number of laboratory studies. The malignant cells of Hodgkin's disease appear to have immunoregulatory effects on T lymphocytes resulting in reduction in their ability to make coordinated immune responses, although their numbers in involved lymph nodes and spleens have been reported to be increased. This contrasts with studies of peripheral blood in Hodgkin's disease, where the absolute number of T lymphocytes has been reported to be decreased, although this is not a consistent finding in all patients. These findings suggest T lymphocytes may be removed from the blood to localize in involved tissues. Serum immunoglobulins are usually normal or increased and therefore B cell function appears to be intact in Hodgkin's patients, at least in the initial phases of their illness. Various authors have suggested that RS cells are derived from T cells, B cells, histiocytes, interdigitating reticulum cells, granulocytes, or undefined cells. The evidence gathered to date is conclusive that RS and Hodgkin (H) cells are *not* derived from immunoregulatory T lymphocyte (helper or suppressor) subsets since they do not form s-ER or react with anti-T cell antibodies.

Although a few investigators have reported finding monoclonal Ig in RS cells, most have found polyclonal Ig, especially IgG (Fig. 10). In order to classify Reed-Sternberg and Hodgkin cells as B lymphoid in origin, these cells would have to break the rule that any B cell and its progeny synthesize only one type of light chain. Despite their morphological similarities to B-immunoblasts, RS cells do not possess the internal structures required to synthesize significant quantities of immunoglobulin, and there is excellent laboratory evidence that these cells possess receptors for the Fc end of the IgG molecule (FcγR) and are able to bind and internalize IgG selectively. The evidence is, on the whole, against a B cell origin for RS and H cells.

Another theory is that the Hodgkin and Reed-Sternberg cells are malignant macrophages or histiocytes. Support for this hypothesis comes from (1) light microscopic similarities of H cells to histiocytes, (2) demonstration of lysozyme and nonspecific esterase in H cells by some researchers, (3) presence of polyclonal IgG within H cells, and

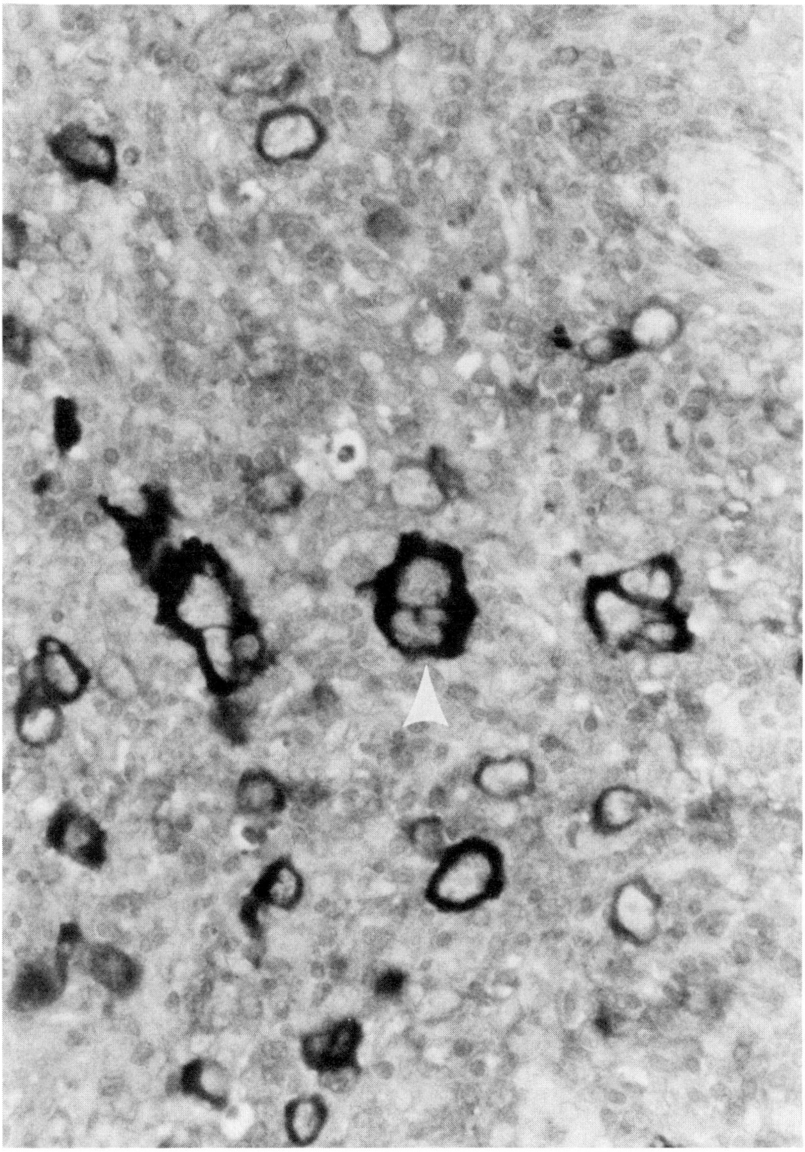

Figure 10: In Hodgkin's disease, immunoperoxidase staining demonstrates presence of large quantities of IgG within numerous Reed-Sternberg and Hodgkin cells (→). Presence of both kappa and lambda light chains indicates the polyclonal origin of the IgG. Phagocytosis of plasma IgG is the most likely explanation for its presence in these malignant cells. Laboratory studies have failed to demonstrate synthesis of IgG by Reed-Sternberg or Hodgkin cells. (Magnification = ×195)

(4) presence of other protein markers for histiocyte in H cells, fibronectin in particular.

Drawbacks to the histiocyte theory are significant, however. The lysozyme findings have been variable from report to report. Examination of RS and H cells by electron microscopy has revealed that these cells lack the cellular organelles associated with phagocytosis, the phagolysosomes that are numerous in macrophages, leading to some doubt whether the RS and H cells can be derived from those cells. Certain receptors normally present on macrophages are absent on R-S and H cells while others not characteristic of macrophages are present, including a human T lymphocyte receptor which is not specific for a given T cell subset. C_3 receptors, regularly present on both macrophages and B lymphocytes, are absent on RS cells. Despite these shortcomings, the macrophage remains in consideration as the progenitor of R-S and H cells, but another candidate cell has recently made considerable inroads on the macrophage theory.

This recently proposed candidate for the cell origin of the RS and H cells is the interdigitating reticulum cell (IRC) of the lymph node paracortex. The functions of this cell are not well understood at present, but it appears to have an influence on the localization of T lymphocytes in the paracortex. These cells are morphologically similar to RS and H cells in that they have great nuclear irregularity and broad irregular cytoplasmic processes. Cytochemical similarities have shown that both IRC and Hodgkin cells possess weak acid phosphatase and nonspecific esterase activity. Functional markers of the IRC are not well established at present, and thus evidence relating RS cells to IRC is still inconclusive. Studies indicate both IRC and RS cells are strongly positive for Ia antigen and react with OKT 4 ⊕ (helper T phenotype) lymphocytes. Ia is a membrane antigen found on a large number of hematopoietic cells including B lymphocytes, "activated" T lymphocytes, monocytes/macrophages, and granulocytes. Ia is also expressed very strongly on the dendritic reticulum cells of the germinal center which is equivalent to the B lymphoid zone of the IRC.

Yet another theory of the origin of the malignant cells of Hodgkin's disease comes from Germany where Stein et al. reported evidence that Hodgkin and RS cells were derived from granulocytic precursors rather than lymphocytes, macrophages, or IRC. These authors developed an antiserum against a Hodgkin's-derived cell line which reacted specifically with RS and H cells but failed to react with any cells of normal tonsil including lymphocytes, macrophages, and IRC. This antiserum did react with normal granulocytic series cells, both mature and immature. Further absorptions with acute myelocytic leukemia (AML) cells removed reactivity to early granulocytic cells but left intact reactivity with neutrophils and H and RS cells. These same authors reported that monoclonal antibodies prepared against certain acute myelo-monocytic leukemia cells cross-reacted with H and RS cells, particularly in nodular sclerosis, mixed cellularity, and lymphocyte-depletion types. The authors suggested that H and RS cells are more closely related to cells of the granulocytic lineage than to any other type of hemato-lymphoid cell.

The large number of studies, many of which contain conflicting data, the uncertainty as to the origin of the malignant cell of Hodgkin's disease, and the histological heterogeneity of the disease make immunopathological studies of cases of Hodgkin's extremely interesting but quite difficult to interpret because there are no confirmed disease-specific markers at this time. Suspension and tissue section immunological marker studies may be useful to perform in the workup of a patient suspected to have Hodgkin's disease because the differential diagnosis often includes B cell type non-Hodgkin's lymphomas which often can be unequivocally identified by these techniques. Distinction between peripheral T cell NHL and Hodgkin's disease is more difficult. Immunological marker studies have identified a predominance of OKT 4 ⊕ "helper" lymphocytes in nodes involved by both HD and peripheral T cell lymphomas. However, the atypical mononuclear variant cells and RS cells often contain polyclonal IgG (both κ and λ light chains present) while in peripheral T cell lymphoma the large mononuclear cells are T cells (s-ER positive).

Atypical reactive lymphoid hyperplasias may also be difficult to separate from Hodgkin's disease by *morphology* alone since both may demonstrate a mixed population of lymphocytes, macrophages, plasma cells, eosinophils, and large "immunoblast-like" cells. The identification of polyvalent IgG in the "immunoblast-like" cells is suggestive of the diagnosis of Hodgkin's disease, while a population of reactive B immunoblasts will contain only one heavy and one light chain of immunoglobulin and a "T" immunoblast should form s-ER and/or react with T cell antibodies.

Conclusion

Most malignant lymphomas have characteristic immunopathological features that can significantly add to the certainty of the morphological diagnosis and thereby improve our ability to predict the prognosis and to select the appropriate therapy for the patient. Benign reactive hyperplasia and pseudolymphomas can be identified with greater certainty with immunological characterization than is possible with morphological examination alone, thus resolving difficult diagnostic problems.

Selected Reading

Aisenberg, A.C.: Current concepts in immunology: Cell-surface markers in lymphoproliferative disease. *N. Engl. J. Med.* 304:331–336, 1981.

Aisenberg, A.C., Block, K., Wilkes, B.M.: Malignant lymphoma with dual B and T cell markers. *J. Exp. Med.* 154:1709–1714.

Beckstead, J., Warnke, R., Bainton, D.: Histochemistry of Hodgkin's disease. *Cancer Treatment Rep.* 66:609–613, 1982.

Berard, C.W., Greene, M.H., Jaffe, E.S., et al.: A multidisciplinary approach to non-Hodgkin's lymphomas. *Ann. Intern. Med.* 94:218–235, 1981.

Black, R.B., et al.: Lymphocyte subpopulations in human lymph nodes: A normal range. *Lymphology* 13:86–90, 1980.

Bloomfield, C.D., Gajl-Peczalska, K.J., Frizzera, G., et al.: Clinical utility of lymphocyte surface markers combined with the Lukes-Collins histologic classification in adult lymphoma. *N. Engl. J. Med.* 301:512–518, 1979.

Bollum, F.J.: Terminal deoxynucleotidyl transferase as a hematopoietic cell marker. *Blood* 54:1203–1215, 1979.

Borowitz, M.J., Croker, B.P., Metzgar, R.S.: Comparison of histologic and immunologic heterogeneity of non-Hodgkin's lymphoma. *Am. J. Path.* 105:97–106, 1981.

Burke, J.S., Butler, J.J.: Malignant lymphoma with a high content of epithelioid histiocytes (Lennert's lymphoma). *Am. J. Clin. Pathol.* 66:1–9, 1976.

Collins, R.D., Waldron, J.A., Glick, A.D.: Results of multiparameter studies of T cell lymphoid neoplasms. *Am. J. Clin. Pathol.* 72:699–707, 1979.

Cossman, J., Berard, C.W.: Malignant lymphomas: The role of immunologic markers in diagnosis, subclassification, and management. *Hum. Pathol.* 11:309–311, 1981.

Edelson, R.D.: Cutaneous T cell lymphoma: Mycosis fungoides, Sezary syndrome, and other variants. *J. Am. Acad. Dermatol.* 2:89–106, 1980.

Foon, K.A., Schroff, R.W., Gale, R.P.: Surface markers on leukemia and lymphoma cells: Recent advances. *Blood* 60:1–19, 1982.

Foucar, K., Goeken, J.A.: Clinical applications of immunological techniques to the diagnosis of lymphoproliferative and immunodeficiency disorders. *Lab. Med.* 13:403–413, 1982.

Garvin, A., Spicer, S., et al.: Immunochemical demonstration of IgG in Reed-Sternberg and other cells in Hodgkin's disease. *J. Exp. Med.* 139:1077–1083, 1974.

Hansen, N., Karle, H.: The elusive Hodgkin's cell. *Scand. J. Haematol.* 26:353–358, 1981.

Harris, N.L., Data, R.E.: The distribution of neoplastic and normal B lymphoid cells in nodular lymphoma. *Hum. Pathol.* 13:610–617, 1982.

Kadin, M., Stites, D., Levy, R., et al.: Exogenous immunoglobulin and the macrophage origin of Reed-Sternberg cells in Hodgkin's disease. *N. Engl. J. Med.* 299:1208–1214, 1978.

Knapp, W. (ed.): *Leukemia Markers: Proceedings of the Leukemia Marker Conference.* London, Academic Press, 1981.

Knowles, D.M., Halper, J.P.: Human T cell malignancies. *Am. J. Path.* 106:187–203, 1982.

Knowles, D.M., Halper, J.P., Jakobiec, F.A.: The immunologic characterization of 40 extranodal lymphoid infiltrates. *Cancer* 49:2321–2335, 1982.

Lennart, K., Kaiserling, D., Muller-Heimelink, H.: *Malignant Lymphomas: Models of Differentiation and Cooperation of Lymphoreticular Cells in Differentiation of Normal and Neoplastic Hematopoietic Cells.* Cold Springs Harbor Conferences on Cell Proliferation, V.5, pp. 897–914, 1978.

Mann, R.B., Jaffe, E.S., Berard, C.W.: Malignant lymphomas—A conceptual understanding of morphologic diversity. *Am. J. Pathol.* 94:105–175, 1979.

Palutke, M., Schnitzer, B., Mirchandani, I., et al.: Increased numbers of lymphocytes with single class surface immunoglobulin in reactive hyperplasia of lymphoid tissue. *Am. J. Clin. Pathol.* 78:316–323, 1982.

Payne, W.V., et al.: Macrophage origin of Reed-Sternberg cells: An immunohistochemical study. *J. Clin. Pathol.* 35:159–166, 1982.

Pinkus, G.S., Said, J.W.: Characterization of non-Hodgkin's lymphomas using multiple cell markers. *Am. J. Pathol.* 94:349–376, 1979.

Poppema, S., et al.: In situ immunologic characterization of cellular constituents in lymph nodes and spleen involved by Hodgkin's disease. *Blood* 59:226–232, 1982.

Saraga, P., Hurlimann, J., Ozzello, L.: Lymphomas and pseudolymphomas of the alimentary tract. *Hum. Pathol.* 12:713–723, 1981.

Stein, J., et al.: Immunohistochemical analysis of the organization of normal lymphoid tissue and non-Hodgkin's lymphomas. *J. Histochem. Cytochem.* 28:746–760, 1980.

Stein, H., et al.: Immunohistological analysis of Hodgkin's and Sternberg-Reed cells. *J. Cancer Res. Clin. Oncol.* 101:125–134, 1981.

Taylor, C.R.: Results of multiparameter studies of B cell lymphomas. *Am. J. Clin. Pathol.* 72:687–698, 1979.

Tubbs, R.R., Sheibani, K., Weiss, R.A., et al.: Tissue immunomicroscopic evaluation of monoclonality of B cell lymphomas. *Am. J. Clin. Pathol.* 76:24–28, 1981.

Van den Tweel, J.G. (ed.): *Malignant Lymphoproliferative Diseases.* The Hague. Leiden Univ. Press, 1980.

Waldron, J.A., Leech, J.J., Glick, A.D., et al.: Malignant lymphoma of peripheral T lymphocyte origin. *Cancer* 40:1604–1617, 1977.

Warnke, R., Levy, R.: Immunopathology of follicular lymphomas: A model of B lymphocyte homing. *N. Engl. J. Med.* 298:481–486, 1978.

Warnke, R., Miller, R., Grogan, T., et al.: Immunologic phenotype in 30 patients with diffuse large-cell lymphoma. *N. Engl. J. Med.* 303:293–300, 1980.

Ziegler, J.L.: Burkitt's lymphoma. *N. Engl. J. Med.* 305:735–744, 1981.

3

Evaluating the Patient with Lymphoma

James O. Armitage, M.D.

Introduction

By far, the most important issue in the evaluation of a patient suspected of having lymphoma is to make sure that the patient does, in fact, have a lymphoma. Although this may sound trite, it most certainly is not. The pathological diagnosis of Hodgkin's disease and the non-Hodgkin's lymphomas is difficult. It is particularly important that a pathologist who is an expert in lymphoma diagnosis has seen the tissue before the clinician initiates therapy. There are certain clues that should alert the clinician to the possibility that the pathological diagnosis of lymphoma might be incorrect. Among the most frequent of these are the diagnosis of extranodal Hodgkin's disease (for example, Hodgkin's disease beginning in the gastrointestinal tract) or the diagnosis of an unusual subtype of non-Hodgkin's lymphoma (such as nodular well-differentiated lymphocytic non-Hodgkin's lymphoma).

Once the clinician has confidence in the histopathological diagnosis of lymphoma, further evaluation is greatly aided by knowledge of the natural history and usual sites of involvement of the various subtypes of lymphomas (Table 1). The relatively predictable pattern of spread of Hodgkin's disease has made possible a reasonably uniform staging evaluation as described below. The non-Hodgkin's lymphomas vary considerably in their usual patterns of involvement. The indolent non-Hodgkin's lymphomas, exemplified by nodular poorly differentiated lymphocytic non-Hodgkin's lymphoma, rarely display systemic symptoms (i.e., fevers, night sweats, or weight loss), and are at least Stage III 90% or more of the time (see Fig. 1). They often

Table 1
Major Clinical Subgroups of Lymphomas

1. Hodgkin's disease
2. Aggressive non-Hodgkin's Lymphomas
   a. diffuse histiocytic
   b. diffuse undifferentiated
   c. diffuse mixed
   d. diffuse poorly differentiated lymphocytic
   e. nodular histiocytic
   f. lymphoblastic lymphoma
3. Indolent non-Hodgkin's Lymphomas
   a. diffuse well-differentiated lymphocytic
   b. nodular poorly differentiated lymphocytic
   c. nodular mixed

involve the bone marrow, liver, and mesenteric lymph nodes and rarely have an extranodal site of presentation. Another indolent non-Hodgkin's lymphoma, diffuse well-differentiated lymphocytic non-Hodgkin's lymphoma, is closely akin to chronic lymphocytic leukemia (i.e., it can be thought of as the tissue manifestation of chronic lymphocytic leukemia) and particularly frequently involves the bone marrow. In contrast with the indolent non-Hodgkin's lymphomas, the aggressive non-Hodgkin's lymphomas, exemplified by diffuse histiocytic lymphoma, frequently cause systemic symptoms, frequently have extranodal sites of presentation, generally do not involve the liver and bone marrow, and are localized (i.e., Stage I or Stage II) at presentation approximately one-third of the time. Thus it is easy to see that a firm histopathological diagnosis and knowledge of the natural history of the particular subtype of lymphoma increase the likelihood of an efficient and accurate staging evaluation.

Before proceeding, it is worthwhile to stop and consider the concept of "staging" cancer. General acceptance of this concept is reasonably new in medicine and its appearance has been the key to intelligent treatment planning. One definition of staging is "to estimate the extent of a malignancy so as to allow an accurate prognosis and intelligent treatment planning." There are, then, three goals of staging. The first is to identify the extent of the patient's disease. In the case of lymphomas, this generally means the anatomical sites of involvement. Table 2 outlines the rules for applying the Ann Arbor staging system that was designed for Hodgkin's disease but is used for all lymphomas in adults. It is of note that this system does not apply equally well to the non-Hodgkin's lymphomas. For example, since

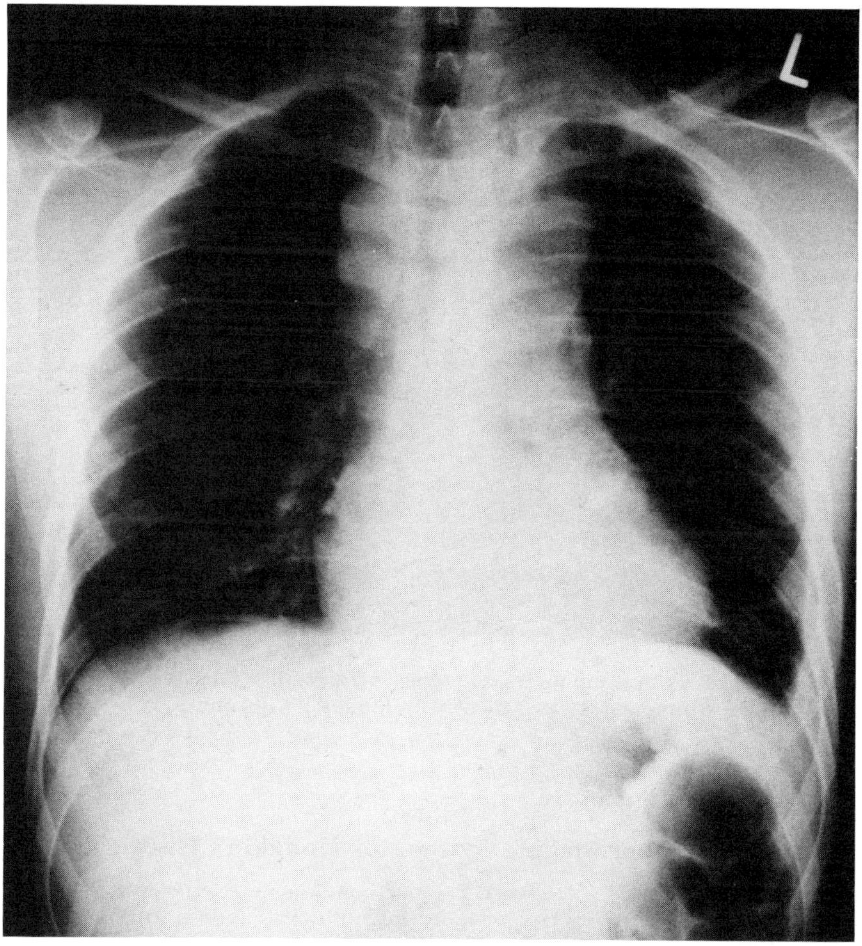

Figure 1A: Prominent mediastinal adenopathy in a patient with Hodgkin's disease.

almost all diffuse well-differentiated lymphocytic non-Hodgkin's lymphomas have bone marrow involvement, they are almost always Stage IV. The tendency for widespread involvement of the other indolent non-Hodgkin's lymphomas makes the Ann Arbor system almost equally unhelpful in nodular poorly differentiated lymphocytic non-Hodgkin's lymphoma and nodular mixed lymphocytic-histiocytic non-Hodgkin's lymphoma. There are other illnesses where staging systems have been developed that do not depend on anatomical extent of the disease. The Rai staging system in chronic lymphocytic

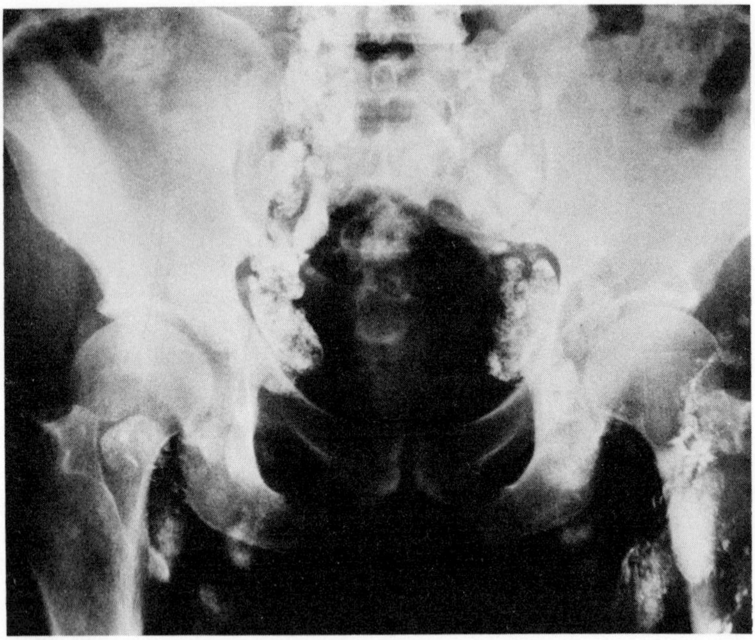

Figure 1B: Lymphangiogram showing enlarged, foamy pelvic and retroperitoneal lymph nodes in a patient with Hodgkin's disease.

Table 2
Ann Arbor Staging System for Hodgkin's Disease

Stage I*	Restricted to one lymph node-bearing area
Stage II*	Two or more areas of nodal involvement on one side of the diaphragm
Stage III*	Lymphatic involvement on both sides of the diaphragm
Stage IV	Liver, bone marrow, or other extensive, extranodal disease
Symptom Status A	Absence of fevers, sweats, or weight loss
Symptom Status B	Unexplained fevers >38°C, drenching night sweats, weight loss of >10% in preceding 6 months
Clinical Stage	The assigned stage based only on history, physical findings, and laboratory and radiologic studies
Pathologic Stage	The assigned stage based only on areas of biopsy proven involvement
Substage E	Localized, extranodal disease

* The spleen and Waldeyer's ring are considered a nodal and not an extranodal disease.

leukemia (Table 3) has functional as well as anatomical designations. The Ann Arbor system also applies less well to the aggressive non-Hodgkin's lymphomas than to Hodgkin's disease because of the frequency of extranodal sites of origin. This is somewhat taken into account by the E designation for extranodal sites of disease, but its application is often awkward. For example, a patient with diffuse histiocytic lymphoma who has a lytic lesion in the femur and also has periaortic and mesenteric lymph node involvement might be called Stage II E or IV, depending upon the observer.

In addition to determining extent of disease, a staging system, to be maximally helpful, needs to give the physician information that allows communication of prognosis to the patient. Different stages should have different responses to therapy or differences in ultimate outcome. With the exceptions noted above, this is generally true with the application of the Ann Arbor staging system to the lymphomas. Finally, and perhaps most importantly, a staging system needs to help the physician choose among available therapies for the disease. The various treatment modalities available to treat cancer (i.e., surgery, radiation therapy, and chemotherapy) are not equally applicable to patients with localized and disseminated disease. Patients with localized disease are candidates for surgery or traditional radiation therapy, while patients with disseminated disease are generally treated with chemotherapy or total body irradiation. In practice, patients with Stage I and sometimes Stage II and III lymphomas are treated with radiation therapy while patients with Stage IV lymphomas and sometimes Stage II and III lymphomas are treated with chemotherapy.

The great majority of patients with Hodgkin's disease and indolent non-Hodgkin's lymphomas and many patients with aggressive non-Hodgkin's lymphomas present with peripheral lymph node enlargement and are diagnosed by the biopsy of a cervical, supraclavicular, or axillary lymph node. A complete history and physical examination will in many cases yield complaints suggesting other sites

Table 3
Rai Staging System in Chronic Lymphocytic Leukemia

Stage	*Characteristics*
0	Lymphocytosis in blood and marrow
1	Lymphadenopathy
2	Splenomegaly and/or hepatomegaly
3	Anemia
4	Thrombocytopenia

of involvement. Sometimes the discovery of lymph nodes on the opposite side of the diaphragm will lead to biopsy and quick documentation of disseminated disease. When no other disease is immediately obvious, the evaluation of the patient should proceed with special attention to the lungs (easily evaluated by a chest roentgenogram), the bone marrow (easily evaluated by a bone marrow biopsy), and the abdominal and retroperitoneal contents (not easily evaluated at all). How to determine involvement in the latter sites is generally the major difficulty encountered in staging patients for lymphoma and will be dealt with below for each of the individual subtypes. Staging patients with extranodal presentation of the aggressive non-Hodgkin's lymphomas, particularly if the diagnosis is made at laparotomy, is a somewhat different problem, but in general the same techniques are used.

The specific applications of the available staging tests and procedures to the various subtypes of the lymphomas will be discussed in the following paragraphs. It is important to remember that there is no absolute consensus regarding the "best" way to accomplish staging evaluation in patients with lymphomas. Although being objective is the goal, it is likely that some of my prejudices will show through.

Hodgkin's Disease

Hodgkin's disease, of all the lymphomas, has a predictable pattern of spread from one lymphatic region to another and tends to involve extranodal sites, other than by direct extension from lymph nodes, only late in the disease. A discovery of the principles of the pattern of spread of Hodgkin's disease was largely the result of studies done at Stanford University by Dr. Henry Kaplan and co-workers. This knowledge has made the evaluation and therapeutic decisions in patients with Hodgkin's disease somewhat standardized. From a practical point of view, when one sets out to stage a patient with Hodgkin's disease, one is looking for reasons to administer chemotherapy rather than radiation therapy and tries to accomplish this by doing the least morbid studies first and proceeding with more difficult tests when the easier ones are not helpful. As noted above, the greatest difficulty comes in determining the presence or absence of intraabdominal or retroperitoneal Hodgkin's disease. The possible methods of evaluation and their appropriate application are described below in the sections on historical evaluation, physical examination, laboratory studies, radiological evaluations, and surgical staging.

Medical History

As is true with most illnesses, a carefully taken history is key to the appropriate evaluation of patients with Hodgkin's disease. Ascertaining the pace of the illness might give some insight into the aggressiveness with which therapy should be pursued. Hodgkin's disease varies from, on one extreme, an indolent but recurring disease with which the patient lives for many years with only minimal therapy to a fulminant disease, particularly likely in older patients, leading to rapid death unless prompt intervention is undertaken. No matter what the pace of the illness, Hodgkin's disease is ultimately fatal unless an accurate evaluation leads to the institution of therapy appropriate to the extent of the disease.

One of the most important aspects of taking a history in patients with Hodgkin's disease is the careful determination of the presence or absence of systemic or "B" systems. These include unexplained fever of greater than 38°C, night sweats, or loss of greater than 10% body weight in the preceding 6 months. Determination of the presence or absence of fever is the most objective, and evaluation to rule out infectious causes of fever is usually sufficient to be confident of the presence of this B symptom. The most subjective evaluation is that of the presence or absence of night sweats. It is important to remember that night sweats in this context refer to drenching sweats and not to a patient being damp around the neck from time to time. Useful questions in this regard include whether or not the patient has to frequently change their night clothes, whether they can wring water out of them, or whether some maneuver to protect the mattress on which they sleep (such as a plastic cover under the sheets) has been implemented by the patient's spouse. Despite a clear definition, it is not always easy to determine whether or not a patient has the systemic symptom of weight loss. The most frequent causes for uncertainty occur in patients who have been dieting and in establishing just what the patient really did weigh several months ago. Despite the imprecision inherent in assigning the patient to symptom status A or B, the assignment is useful and important. In Hodgkin's disease and the aggressive non-Hodgkin's lymphomas, it has tremendous prognostic significance.

Pruritus was formally considered a B symptom, but lack of definite evidence for its effect on prognosis has led to its exclusion. Generalized or sometimes localized pruritus is a frequent companion of Hodgkin's disease. The mechanism leading to pruritus, as with the mechanism leading to other systemic symptoms, is not known for certain. However, the presence of generalized pruritus can be a hint to the diagnosis of Hodgkin's disease and to its recurrence after apparently successful therapy.

One clear goal of history taking in patients with Hodgkin's disease should be an attempt to ascertain whether or not there are sites of involvement beyond those already known. The presence of a swollen face and eyelids on arising in the morning should suggest superior vena caval obstruction. Shortness of breath would suggest thoracic involvement by Hodgkin's disease, and a cough on reclining suggests a pleural effusion. Pain involving any site in the body can be a symptom that leads to appropriate roentgenographic studies and biopsy to document advanced stage disease. Particular examples of this might be bone pain resulting from osseous involvement by the disease, back pain because of retroperitoneal lymphadenopathy, or back pain and neurologic dysfunction suggestive of epidural disease.

One unusual symptom which, although it occurs infrequently, has raised considerable interest is pain at a site of involvement by Hodgkin's disease associated with ethanol ingestion. The exact mechanism of this occurrence is uncertain, but on occasion it can lead to the discovery of previously unsuspected sites of involvement.

Physical Examination

Careful physical examination is important in evaluation of patients with Hodgkin's disease. Detection of scleral icterus can be the first clue to intrinsic hepatic or extrahepatic nodal disease. However, it is worthwhile to remember that occasional patients with Hodgkin's disease may be jaundiced with no involvement anywhere near the liver. Hepatic dysfunction can, on rare occasions, be the result of a distant effect of the Hodgkin's disease on the liver which disappears when the disease is effectively treated. A careful examination of lymph node-bearing areas is vital in the evaluation of a patient with Hodgkin's disease. The status of preauricular, anterior and posterior cervical, supraclavicular, subclavicular, epitrochlear, axillary, and inguinal lymph nodes should all be carefully ascertained. Lymph nodes involved by Hodgkin's disease characteristically have a firm, rubbery texture. The occurrence of large lymph nodes and the texture of palpable lymph nodes are not sufficient, however, to diagnose Hodgkin's disease, and if therapy would be affected by involvement at a particular site, a biopsy should be done.

Cutaneous involvement by Hodgkin's disease is rare but should be looked for. Examination of the chest might reveal asymmetric dullness suggestive of pleural effusions. Abdominal examination should be directed towards the presence or absence of hepatomegaly, splenomegaly, or abdominal masses. A complete examination should be done for unusual but potentially important manifestations of Hodgkin's disease.

Laboratory Evaluation

The hematological evaluation in patients with Hodgkin's disease is frequently abnormal and occasionally important in determining the extent of involvement. The extent of hematological abnormalities in a general way reflects the extent of disease. That is, patients with advanced disease are more likely to have abnormal blood counts than patients with localized, asymptomatic disease. The white blood cell count in patients with Hodgkin's disease is typically normal or slightly increased. The differential white blood cell count typically shows a decreased number of lymphocytes and occasionally an increase in neutrophils and/or eosinophils. An increase in the absolute number of lymphocytes would be extremely unusual in Hodgkin's disease. Patients with advanced Hodgkin's disease are frequently anemic. The anemia is usually normocytic and normochromic as seen in the "anemia of chronic disease." Other mechanisms for anemia that should be considered include marrow replacement, blood loss from gastrointestinal disease (extremely infrequent in Hodgkin's disease), and marrow suppression following therapy. A platelet count in Hodgkin's disease is typically normal or increased. Thrombocytosis is, of course, found in patients who have had a splenectomy as part of their staging evaluation. Thrombocytopenia in a patient with Hodgkin's disease is most likely related to marrow suppression from cytotoxic therapy, marrow replacement, or hypersplenism.

A bone marrow evaluation should be done as part of the staging evaluation in patients with Hodgkin's disease. Although bone marrow involvement is infrequent (occurring in less than 10% of newly diagnosed patients), the examination is safe, easy to perform, and relatively inexpensive. If positive, its implications are profound. The diagnosis of Hodgkin's disease can essentially never be made on a bone marrow aspirate. Adequate bone marrow biopsy specimens, usually obtained with a Jamshidi needle, are essential. The quantity of bone marrow examined will determine the yield in bone marrow examinations in Hodgkin's disease. Bone marrow cores totaling at least 30 mm in length should be available for examination. Whether these come from one very large biopsy specimen, multiple biopsy samples on one posterior iliac crest, or bilateral iliac crest biopsy specimens is less important than the total size of the specimen examined. The diagnosis of Hodgkin's disease in the bone marrow is histologically a difficult one. Whether or not typical Reed-Sternberg cells are necessary to make this diagnosis in a patient with known Hodgkin's disease elsewhere has been a point for debate. It is important to remember that patients with Hodgkin's disease can occasionally have granulomas found in marrow and other organs that not only do not represent involvement by Hodgkin's disease but are associated with a better prognosis than seen in patients who lack these disseminated granulomas.

Routine screening chemistry studies are important in evaluating patients with Hodgkin's disease. While any of these tests can be abnormal (e.g., elevated calcium in patients with extensive bone disease), the most important studies are probably liver and renal function tests. Abnormal liver function studies in patients with Hodgkin's disease suggest, but by no means prove, hepatic involvement. Serum alkaline phosphatase and serum bilirubin levels, in particular, can be elevated in patients with Hodgkin's disease without metastatic spread to the liver. It is extremely important that patients not be classified as Stage IV on the basis of hepatic involvement without biopsy proof of Hodgkin's disease in the liver. Renal studies in patients with Hodgkin's disease are occasionally abnormal because of bilateral ureteral obstruction by retroperitoneal lymphadenopathy. This has urgent therapeutic implications. Occasionally a patient with Hodgkin's disease will have the nephrotic syndrome as a distant effect on Hodgkin's disease on the kidney without renal involvement. Hodgkin's disease very rarely involves the renal parenchyma.

Evaluations of serum proteins in patients with Hodgkin's disease are occasionally abnormal but rarely helpful in assigning stage. Patients with advanced disease may have hypoalbuminemia. Elevation of "reactive" proteins (e.g., fibrinogen) is presumably the mechanism that leads to an elevated sedimentation rate in some patients. Patients with advanced Hodgkin's disease, particularly with liver involvement, will occasionally have increased gamma globulins. Monoclonal gammopathies are very unusual in Hodgkin's disease.

Patients with Hodgkin's disease almost uniformly have alterations in immune function. This is most profound in patients with advanced, symptomatic disease but can also be identified in patients with localized disease. Abnormalities that have been identified include alterations in lymphocyte numbers and subpopulations, altered in vitro lymphocyte responsiveness, decreased skin test responsiveness and, in some cases, total anergy. These alterations in immune function seem to be lifelong in many patients cured of Hodgkin's disease. Whether they represent abnormalities in the patient that lead to acquiring Hodgkin's disease, an effect of the disease itself, or, in the case of patients who have been previously treated, the effect of therapy, is not clear. It does seem certain that altered immune function is an important contributor to the frequent deaths from infection seen in patients with Hodgkin's disease.

A number of miscellaneous laboratory studies have been noted to be abnormal in patients with Hodgkin's disease. Perhaps the most interesting of these is the test for serum copper. Following the serum copper level has been suggested as a useful test to monitor the activity of Hodgkin's disease. Elevated serum copper levels are found typically in patients with active disease and normal serum copper levels in patients who are cured or in remission.

Radiological and Radionuclide Evaluation

The intrathoracic region is the most frequent site of involvement by Hodgkin's disease in which radiological evaluation is important. The chest roentgenogram, which should be done on every patient with Hodgkin's disease, frequently will show mediastinal and/or hilar adenopathy (Fig. 1A). This is particularly characteristic for young females with the nodular sclerosing histological variety of Hodgkin's disease. The extent of intrathoracic involvement by Hodgkin's disease has important therapeutic implications. Patients with extremely large mediastinal masses (i.e., those occupying greater than one-third of the transthoracic diameter) have a high risk of recurrence after treatment with radiation therapy alone and are frequently treated with chemotherapy, with or without concomitant radiation. When radiation alone is chosen to treat Hodgkin's disease, it is important that the extent of intrathoracic disease be known as precisely as possible. This requires the use of computerized axial tomographic (CAT) scans or whole lung tomograms. It is not unusual for localized extranodal extension of Hodgkin's disease in the lung parenchyma to be missed on the chest roentgenogram. This could mean that Hodgkin's disease would be excluded from the radiation treatment portal and thus guarantee recurrence.

The other extremely important radiological evaluation is that for the determination of the extent of intraabdominal and particularly retroperitoneal involvement. Studies available for this purpose include bipedal lymphangiography, CAT scan, abdominal ultrasound, gallium scan, intravenous pyelogram, liver-spleen scan, and gastrointestinal contrast roentgenograms. Not all abdominal and retroperitoneal structures are equally likely to be involved by Hodgkin's disease. While retroperitoneal nodes frequently contain Hodgkin's disease, mesenteric lymph nodes do so only rarely. The spleen and liver are commonly involved by Hodgkin's disease, but the intestinal tract and kidneys are rarely involved. The choice of appropriate radiological and isotope studies must take these facts into consideration. Retroperitoneal lymph nodes can be evaluated with the lymphangiogram, CAT scan, abdominal ultrasound, intravenous pyelogram, or gallium scan (Table 4). Of these studies the most experience is available with bipedal lymphangiography. Lymphangiograms are very accurate in determining involvement of visualized retroperitoneal lymph nodes (Fig. 1B). They have the advantage of revealing characteristics of the internal architecture of lymph nodes, in addition to their size and position. Lymphangiograms in Hodgkin's disease are rarely falsely negative (approximately 5–10%) and a positive test has a high likelihood (approximately 85%) of detecting involvement of the visualized nodes. The major shortcoming of lymphangiography is that it does not visualize upper abdominal lymph nodes. Abdominal CAT scans offer both advantages and disadvantages when compared with lymphangiography. CAT scans do visualize the upper abdominal structures and give information regarding both the size and texture of the spleen and liver. CAT scans also visualize the intraperitoneal structures and

Table 4
Value of Radiologic and Radionuclide Studies for the Evaluation of the Abdominal and Retroperitoneal Patients with Lymphoma

		Relative Value	
Study	*HD*	*Aggressive NHL*	*Indolent NHL*
Bipedal lymphangiography	+ + +	+ + +	+ + +
CAT scan	+ + +	+ + +	+ + +
Ultrasound	+ + +	+ + +	+ + +
Intravenous pyelography	+ +	+ +	+ +
Gallium scan	+ +	+ +	+
GI series	+	+	+
L-S scan	+	+	+

+ + + often included in initial evaluation, very accurate >75%
+ + of occasional value
+ only in special circumstances, generally not appropriate

thus can identify enlarged mesenteric lymph nodes. However, as was mentioned earlier, mesenteric nodes are rarely involved by Hodgkin's disease. Abdominal ultrasonography, like CAT scans, can visualize all the intraperitoneal and retroperitoneal contents. Although there are some data available to suggest that CAT scans have an accuracy in identifying abdominal Hodgkin's disease similar to that of lymphangiography, very little data are available in the literature regarding the use of ultrasonography. However, when an expert ultrasonographer is available (this procedure is particularly dependent on the skill of the person performing the test), ultrasonography is probably roughly comparable in utility to CAT scans. As a general rule, CAT scans are more useful in obese patients and ultrasonography in particularly slender patients. These three studies, which are the most useful in nonsurgical staging of intraabdominal lymphomas, should be thought of as complementary. In addition to the advantages and disadvantages listed above, safety, cost, and ease of application need to be considered (Table 5). Lymphangiograms are difficult to perform, relatively expensive, and should be used only with caution in older patients because of the risk of respiratory embarrassment. Nevertheless, lymphangiograms are the most accurate test in evaluating retroperitoneal lymphadenopathy and have the added advantage of retention of the dye in the nodes for months which allows reevaluation by repeated abdominal roentgenograms. CAT scans are safe and easy to perform. They are, however, very expensive and do not demonstrate involvement of normal sized nodes. Abdominal ultrasonography is also safe, easy to perform, and relatively inexpensive. Unfortunately, ultrasonography has the least documented accuracy and is the most dependent on the skill of the performer. The decision as to which test, or tests to utilize at any particular institution and for any particular patient must take into account all of these factors.

Table 5
Comparison of the Three Major Studies for Evaluating the Abdomen

	Accuracy	*Economy (lowest cost)*	*Risk*
Lymphangiogram	1	2	1
CAT scan	2	3	3
Ultrasound	3	1	3

1 = most accurate, most economic, lowest risk
2 = intermediate
3 = least accurate, least economic, highest risk

There are a number of other studies that have considerably less utility for the evaluation of intraabdominal Hodgkin's disease. Gallium scans have been rather extensively evaluated in the staging of patients with lymphomas. They are most accurate in Hodgkin's disease and the aggressive non-Hodgkin's lymphomas and least accurate in the indolent non-Hodgkin's lymphomas. Bowel uptake of gallium unfortunately limits its use in detecting intraabdominal lymphomas. Gallium scans are most useful in detecting Hodgkin's disease above the diaphragm or in bone.

Intravenous pyelograms can give indirect evidence of retroperitoneal lymphadenopathy. Their most important use in evaluating patients with Hodgkin's disease is to rule out ureteral compression by retroperitoneal tumor which can be insidious and requires urgent intervention. Gastrointestinal contrast roentgenograms are of very little value in the evaluation of patients with Hodgkin's disease because of the infrequent involvement of the bowel. They should be reserved only for situations where there is a high clinical suspicion of gastrointestinal tract abnormalities.

Liver-spleen scans are of very little use in the evaluation of patients with Hodgkin's disease because of the frequent occurrence of both false negative and false positive scans. One other radionuclide study that can be of value in evaluating some patients with Hodgkin's disease is the bone scan. Bone scans tend to be more accurate than bone roentgenograms in identifying osseous involvement by Hodgkin's disease. However, their use should be reserved for patients with complaints suggestive of bone involvement by the disease.

Surgical Staging

The details of surgical staging in patients with Hodgkin's disease are dealt with in another section in this monograph. However, a few comments about when to utilize surgical staging are appropriate in this section. Surgical staging should be reserved for young patients with no other medical problems that would make laparotomy hazardous (e.g., severe heart disease) and who have not had any findings in nonsurgical staging that would indicate a need for treatment with chemotherapy (e.g., bone marrow involvement). A staging laparotomy is not an obligatory part of staging patients with Hodgkin's disease and should only be performed after careful consideration of its implications for the patient. Many patients with advanced disease will be able to have their stage pathologically documented with procedures other than staging laparotomy. For example, percutaneous or peritoneoscopically directed liver biopsies might demonstrate hepatic involvement without the need for laparotomy.

Indolent Non-Hodgkin's Lymphomas

One could make a very good argument that staging procedures in patients with indolent non-Hodgkin's lymphomas, particularly nodular poorly differentiated lymphocytic non-Hodgkin's lymphoma and diffuse well-differentiated lymphocytic non-Hodgkin's lymphoma, are superfluous. It appears that when extensive staging evaluations are performed (including staging laparotomy), more than 90% of these patients will be Stage III or IV. None of the procedures used in staging will have an accuracy greater than the initial knowledge that 90–95% of patients in question have at least Stage III disease. Because of this, the aggressiveness with which one pursues staging in the indolent non-Hodgkin's lymphomas will depend upon the importance attached to finding a rare patient with localized disease who can be cured with radiation therapy.

Medical History

History taking in indolent non-Hodgkin's lymphomas, as in the other lymphomas, should be directed at eliciting complaints suggestive of involvement of certain anatomical sites by disease, ascertaining the presence or absence of systemic symptoms, and determining the disability that the disease is causing the patient. The latter part is particularly pertinent in the indolent non-Hodgkin's lymphomas. Since these illnesses are associated with a relatively long survival, frequently cause minimal disability, and occasionally undergo spontaneous regression, not all patients need to be treated initially. Careful determination of the implications of the disease for the patient will be helpful in planning subsequent management.

The problems of determining the presence or absence of systemic symptoms are the same in non-Hodgkin's lymphomas as in Hodgkin's disease. However, in the indolent non-Hodgkin's lymphomas, systemic symptoms are relatively unusual, occurring in only 20–30% of patients.

Physical Examination

Typically, the examination of the patient with an indolent non-Hodgkin's lymphoma will reveal an elderly individual with diffuse, nontender lymphadenopathy, and few other findings. The indolent non-Hodgkin's lymphomas, more frequently than other lymphomas, are found to involve the epitrochlear lymph nodes. Involved nodes tend to be firm and rubbery in texture.

A thorough and careful examination will sometimes hint at other sites of involvement. Patients with indolent non-Hodgkin's lymphomas not infrequently have orbital involvement. Waldeyer's ring is more frequently involved in the non-Hodgkin's lymphomas than in Hodgkin's disease. Examination of the chest and abdomen might reveal the signs of a chylous pleural effusion or ascites. Hepatomegaly and splenomegaly are both characteristic of involvement of these organs by indolent non-Hodgkin's lymphomas, and palpable abdominal masses are more frequent in these disorders than in Hodgkin's disease. Swelling of an extremity can be the result of a lymphatic obstruction by tumor. Prostatic involvement in the indolent non-Hodgkin's lymphomas is more common than in other types of lymphomas. Cutaneous and central nervous system involvement are unusual in the indolent non-Hodgkin's lymphomas.

Laboratory Evaluation

Involvement of the peripheral blood in the indolent non-Hodgkin's lymphomas is much more common than in Hodgkin's disease or in the aggressive non-Hodgkin's lymphomas. Elevated white counts due to circulating lymphoma cells are most likely in diffuse well-differentiated lymphocytic lymphoma and nodular poorly differentiated lymphocytic lymphoma. Circulating cleaved, small lymphocytes in the latter disorder have led to this being called "lymphosarcoma cell leukemia" in the past. Anemia is an unusual early finding in the indolent non-Hodgkin's lymphomas. When it does occur, it can reflect massive bone marrow involvement, an autoimmune hemolytic process or, more rarely, blood loss or marrow suppression. Thrombocytopenia on presentation in the indolent non-Hodgkin's lymphomas is most likely due to hypersplenism, marrow replacement, or autoimmune platelet destruction.

The bone marrow is frequently involved in the indolent non-Hodgkin's lymphomas and is seen in approximately 90% of patients with diffuse well-differentiated lymphocytic lymphoma, in approximately 60% of patients with nodular poorly differentiated lymphocytic lymphoma, and in approximately 40% of patients with nodular mixed lymphoma. Marrow involvement, which is much more likely to be detected by marrow biopsy than by examination of aspirate smears, is typically in the form of paratrabecular lymphoid nodules. Diffuse involvement, particularly in the well-differentiated lymphocytic subtype, can occur. As mentioned previously, the chances for detecting bone marrow involvement depends upon the quantity of marrow examined.

Serum chemistry determinations and protein studies will only occasionally be important in assigning stage in the indolent non-Hodgkin's lymphomas. Although more frequent in the aggressive non-Hodgkin's lymphomas, an elevated serum lactic dehydrogenase (LDH) will occasionally reflect tumor mass and serve as a marker for disease activity. Abnormal liver function studies can be a reflection of hepatic involvement by an indolent lymphoma. Unsuspected ureteral compression due to retroperitoneal lymphadenopathy can lead to renal insufficiency. Serum protein electrophoresis will occasionally reveal a monoclonal gammopathy. This is particularly likely in the diffuse well-differentiated lymphocytic lymphomas when plasma cytoid differentiation is evident in the tumor cells. Quantitation of immunoglobulins will frequently reveal low levels.

Immune alterations in the indolent non-Hodgkin's lymphomas, while often present, are typically less severe than seen in Hodgkin's disease and in the aggressive non-Hodgkin's lymphomas. This might partly be related to the lower incidence of systemic symptoms in the indolent non-Hodgkin's lymphomas.

Radiological and Radionuclide Evaluations

Intrathoracic involvement by the indolent non-Hodgkin's lymphomas is much less likely than in Hodgkin's disease. The chest roentgenogram might reveal mediastinal or hilar adenopathy, parenchymal involvement, or pleural effusion, but none of these is the rule. Curative radiotherapy is rarely chosen as the initial treatment in indolent non-Hodgkin's lymphomas, and there is much less need for CAT scans of the thorax or whole lung tomograms to accurately define the extent of the disease.

As in the other lymphomas, evaluation of intraperitoneal and retroperitoneal structures is the major object of radiological evaluation.

Because the indolent non-Hodgkin's lymphomas frequently involve the mesenteric lymph nodes, they potentially pose a different problem from Hodgkin's disease. However, involvement is generally extensive, and the lymphangiogram is still a good predictor of abdominal involvement by the disease. As with Hodgkin's disease, bipedal lymphangiography, CAT scans, and ultrasound are the most useful tests for determining the presence and extent of intraabdominal lymphoma (Table 4). Each has its own advantages and disadvantages and the studies are frequently complementary rather than redundant. A special comment is appropriate regarding the place of intravenous pyelograms in the management of patients with indolent non-Hodgkin's lymphomas. These patients are often followed without therapy for what can be extended periods of time. Thus they are particularly at risk for silent ureteral compression due to retroperitoneal adenopathy. Intravenous pyelograms should be performed intermittently in patients with known retroperitoneal lymphoma while they are being followed without therapy to avoid the catastrophy of silent ureteral compression and renal failure.

Gastrointestinal tract involvement is much more frequent in the non-Hodgkin's lymphomas than in Hodgkin's disease. However, the indolent non-Hodgkin's lymphomas are less likely to involve the gastrointestinal tract than the aggressive non-Hodgkin's lymphomas. Still, particularly in patients with involvement of Waldeyer's ring, upper and lower gastrointestinal contrast roentgenograms will occasionally be appropriate in the evaluation of these patients. This should be done when symptoms or physical findings suggest gastrointestinal tract involvement because of possible therapeutic implications (i.e., associated with the risk of perforation during therapy). The indolent lymphomas do not regularly concentrate gallium and thus gallium scans should not be done. Liver-spleen scans are rarely helpful in patients with indolent non-Hodgkin's lymphomas and should be done only under special circumstances.

Other radiological studies will rarely be necessary or helpful in patients with indolent non-Hodgkin's lymphomas. The most likely to be helpful is a bone scan in patients with complaints or physical findings suggestive of osseous involvement.

Surgical Staging

While some patients with indolent non-Hodgkin's lymphomas will have the diagnosis made at laparotomy, staging laparotomy as part of the evaluation is rarely indicated. These patients tend to be old (median age >60 years) and have other illnesses that make laparotomy hazardous. In addition, other studies, sometimes including percutaneous or peritoneoscopically directed liver biopsy, will document extensive disease in a great majority of patients.

Aggressive Non-Hodgkin's Lymphomas

The aggressive non-Hodgkin's lymphomas are a somewhat diverse group of diseases that have in common a poor natural history but the potential for long-term survival with therapy. As in all the non-Hodgkin's lymphomas, these diseases are more frequent in the elderly, but when non-Hodgkin's lymphomas do occur in children they are usually of the aggressive variety. The approach to patients with diffuse histiocytic lymphoma, the most common of the aggressive non-Hodgkin's lymphomas, will in some instances be different from that appropriate to the less frequent undifferentiated Burkitt's lymphoma or lymphoblastic lymphomas. These differences will be pointed out in the following paragraphs. In addition, aggressive non-Hodgkin's lymphomas (especially diffuse histiocytic lymphoma) have a particular predilection for extranodal presentations. This can lead to an altered staging approach and frequently complicates the application of the Ann Arbor staging system.

Medical History

History taking in patients with aggressive non-Hodgkin's lymphomas should emphasize the same points mentioned in the previous sections for Hodgkin's disease and the indolent non-Hodgkin's lymphomas. It is important to ascertain the pace of the disease. The aggressive non-Hodgkin's lymphomas are frequently rapidly growing and potentially rapidly lethal disorders. The prompt identification of sites of disease and institution of appropriate therapy are imperative. Patients with aggressive non-Hodgkin's lymphomas are more likely to have "B" symptoms than patients with indolent non-Hodgkin's lymphomas. Because of the considerable prognostic significance, careful questioning should ascertain the presence or absence of fevers, night sweats, or weight loss. In addition, patients with aggressive non-Hodgkin's lymphomas frequently complain of pruritus. Identification of a positive relationship of this complaint to the lymphoma can be helpful as recurrence of pruritus often heralds relapse after initially successful therapy.

It is, of course, important to identify potential sites of involvement in order to expedite the staging evaluation. Unlike the indolent non-Hodgkin's lymphomas, the aggressive non-Hodgkin's lymphomas frequently involve extranodal sites. Particularly when dealing with lymphoblastic lymphoma and undifferentiated Burkitt's lymphoma, an attempt should be made to inquire for complaints suggestive of central nervous system disease. The frequency of cardiopulmonary disease, gastrointestinal disease, and bone involvement makes the identification of complaints relating to these and other sites of extranodal disease important.

Physical Examination

The physical examination of a patient with an aggressive non-Hodgkin's lymphoma should be thorough so any otherwise unsuspected sites of disease involvement will be detected. Detection of icterus might be the first hint of hepatic involvement or an associated hemolytic anemia. Abnormalities of extraocular muscle function might be the clue that leads to the diagnosis of meningeal lymphoma. Waldeyer's ring should be carefully examined because of a relatively high frequency of involvement. In dealing with undifferentiated Burkitt's lymphoma, it is important to remember that tumors of the facial bones occur frequently. Diffuse histiocytic lymphoma is the most common lymphoma to involve the thyroid gland. A careful examination of the lymph nodes in all lymph node-bearing sites is vital. Cardiopulmonary examination should be done carefully and might reveal signs suggestive of pleural effusion, superior vena caval obstruction, or even lymphomatous involvement of the heart. Hepatomegaly and/or splenomegaly are relatively frequent. Intraperitoneal or retroperitoneal masses might be palpable. Testicular involvement by these tumors is not rare and should be looked for. Although rectal lymphoma is most unusual, occult blood in the stool might be the first hint of gastrointestinal involvement by the tumor. When patients complain of back pain, a careful neurologic examination might reveal signs of epidural compression by tumor. Finally, cutaneous involvement, particularly in the "T" cell varieties of aggressive non-Hodgkin's lymphomas, is not uncommon.

Laboratory Studies

It is unusual in diffuse histiocytic lymphoma, but not in lymphoblastic or undifferentiated Burkitt's lymphoma, to have circulating tumor cells detected on examination of the peripheral blood smear. Quantitation of the formed elements in the blood might reveal leukopenia resulting from bone marrow involvement, anemia which might have diverse causes including bone marrow involvement, tumor-related gastrointestinal blood loss, anemia related to organ dysfunction (e.g., renal failure) or autoimmune hemolytic anemia, and thrombocytopenia usually related to either marrow involvement or hypersplenism. Examination of the bone marrow should be done in essentially all cases. Except in Burkitt's and lymphoblastic lymphoma, the bone marrow aspirate is unlikely to reveal tumor cells. It is important to have an adequate bone marrow biopsy, but involvement by diffuse histiocytic lymphoma is found only 10–15% of the time.

Routine chemistry studies of liver and renal function studies should be performed and might reveal abnormalities reflecting involvement of those organs by lymphoma. Protein electrophoresis will occasionally reveal a monoclonal protein spike, but it is more likely to be normal or reveal slight hypogammaglobulinemia. An evaluation of the patient's immune status by skin tests or by looking at lymphocyte subpopulations and function will frequently reveal abnormalities, more often in patients with "B" symptoms.

Radiological and Radionuclide Evaluation

All of the aggressive non-Hodgkin's lymphomas can involve the thoracic viscera and produce abnormalities on chest roentgenograms. These are therefore absolutely necessary in these patients' evaluation. Lymphoblastic lymphoma characteristically produces mediastinal masses, particularly in young men (Fig. 2A). Essentially any other abnormality can be seen on the chest roentgenogram in any of these lymphomas. When primary therapy of a tumor of the mediastinum or neck with radiotherapy is being contemplated, CAT scan of the chest or whole lung and mediastinal tomograms should be done to determine carefully the extent of disease.

As with the other lymphomas, radiological evaluation of involvement of the intraperitoneal and retroperitoneal structures is the most difficult aspect. The same tests are of value in the aggressive non-

Hodgkin's lymphomas as in Hodgkin's disease and indolent non-Hodgkin's lymphomas (Table 4). In general, lymphangiography, CAT scans, and abdominal ultrasounds are the most useful studies (Figs. 2B and 2C). The comments from the section on radiological evaluation in Hodgkin's disease generally pertain to the aggressive non-Hodgkin's lymphomas. It is important to remember that these tumors are more likely to involve the gastrointestinal tract than the other subtypes

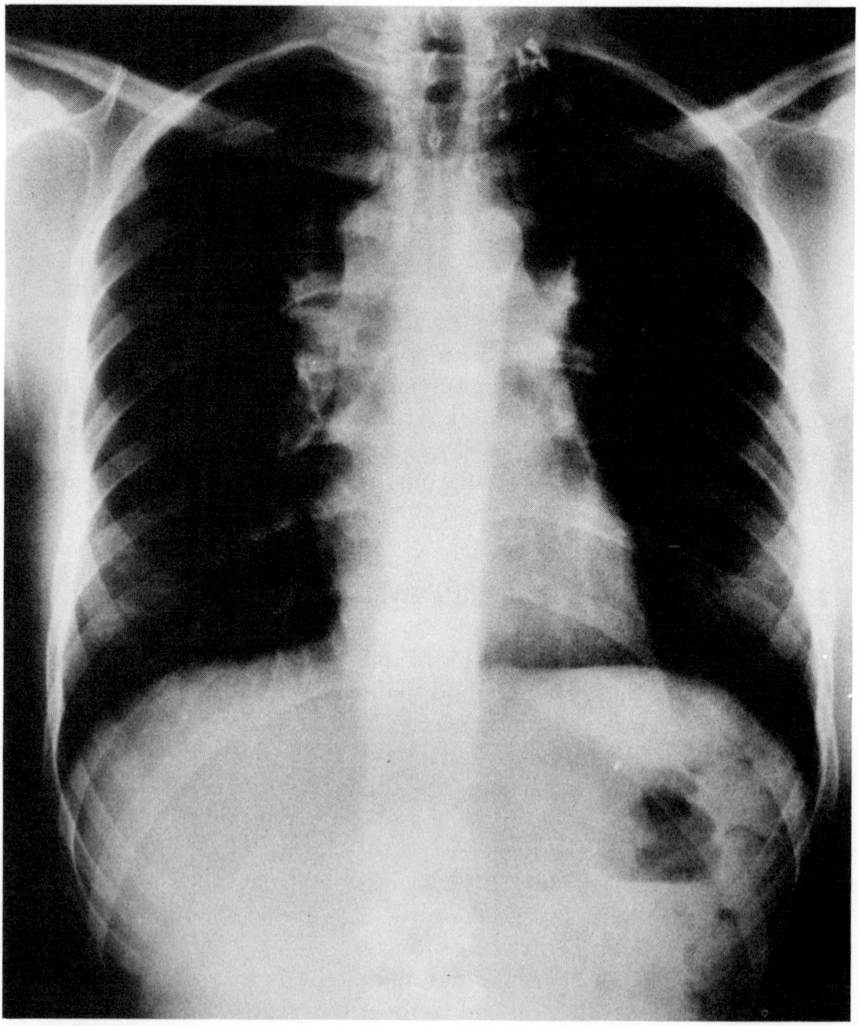

Figure 2A: Mediastinal and hilar adenopathy in a patient with lymphoblastic lymphoma.

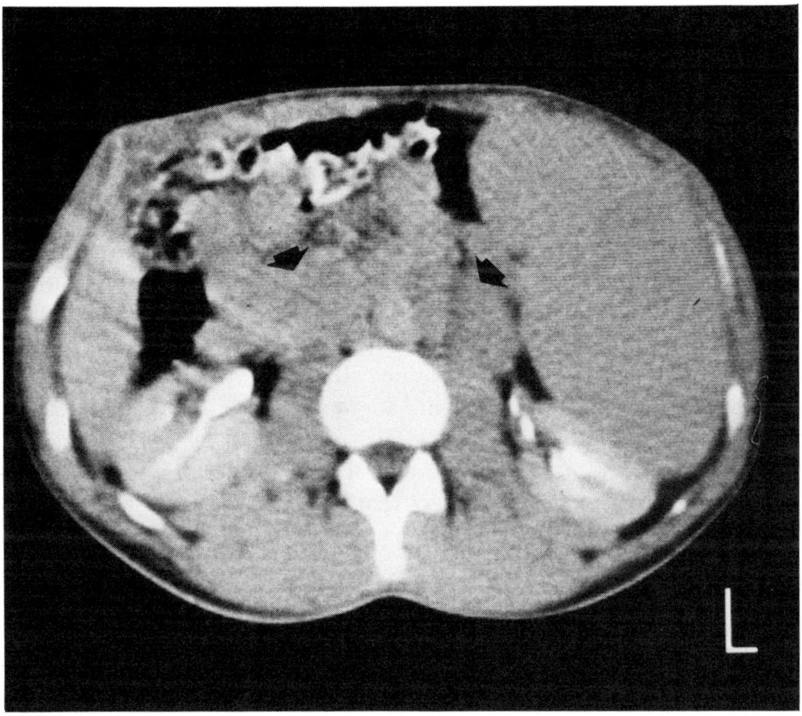

Figure 2B: Abdominal CAT scan showing periaortic adenopathy in a patient with diffuse histiocytic lymphoma.

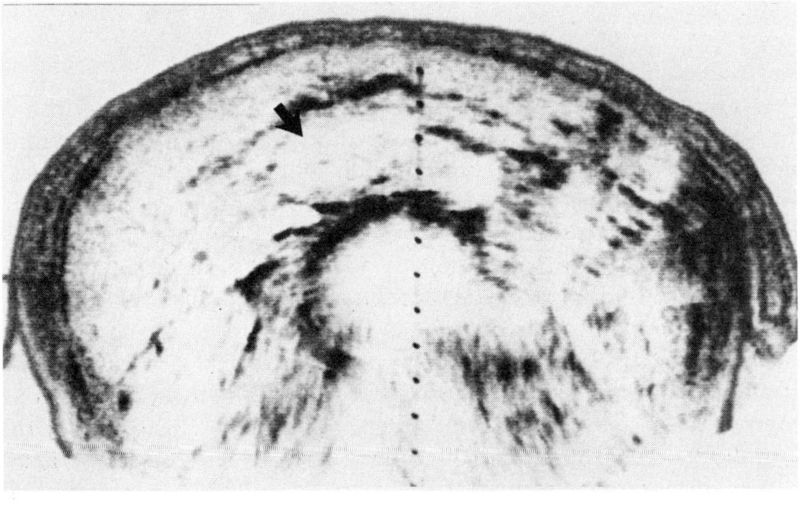

Figure 2C: Abdominal ultrasound showing periaortic adenopathy in a patient with diffuse histiocytic lymphoma.

of lymphomas and thus contrast studies are more likely to be useful and should be done in patients where gastrointestinal tract involvement is suspected. As noted above with the other lymphomas, radionuclide scans are only helpful in a few selected cases.

Surgical Staging

In general, staging laparotomies will rarely be appropriate in the aggressive non-Hodgkin's lymphomas. It is usually possible to document extensive disease in patients with peripheral nodal presentations without doing staging laparotomies. In addition, these patients are generally older and at somewhat higher risk for complications following laparotomy than the typical patient with Hodgkin's disease. However, the frequency of extranodal and intraabdominal presentation of these tumors and the fact that they are localized at diagnosis approximately one-third of the time means that they will frequently be diagnosed during a surgical procedure. It is extremely important that the surgeon who comes upon intraabdominal, aggressive non-Hodgkin's lymphoma at operation performs the appropriate biopsies to document the extent of disease and avoid complicating the patient's later therapy. In addition, resection of gastrointestinal primary tumors can occasionally be curative and can eliminate the risk of perforation with the initiation of effective therapy.

Summary

The majority of patients with lymphomas will present with peripheral lymphadenopathy and have the diagnosis made by lymph node biopsy. Usually the lymph node will have been in the neck, supraclavicular area, or the axilla (Table 6). In many cases, a careful history and physical examination, initial chest roentgenogram, or routine laboratory studies will quickly identify other sites of potential involvement by lymphoma which, after being confirmed by biopsy, will document an advanced stage of disease and lead to the initiation of chemotherapy. If the patient remains in Stage I or II after these studies, a bone marrow biopsy should be done. The chances of positive marrow biopsy will vary greatly depending on the histology of the lymphoma. A positive marrow biopsy will always lead to the institution of systemic therapy. If the marrow biopsy is negative, it is necessary to proceed with further studies looking for disease on the

Table 6
Sequence of Studies in Evaluating a Patient with Lymphoma Presenting with Peripheral Nodes and/or Above Diaphragm Disease

Initial Evaluations 1. History and Physical 2. Chest x-ray 3. Routine Lab Studies 4. Marrow Biopsy	→	If characteristic node or abnormal finding, perform biopsy to prove advanced disease
↓		
If not Stage III or IV do abdominal and retroperitoneal evaluation 1. Lymphangiogram 2. CAT Scan 3. Ultrasound	→	If abnormal treat as advanced disease
↓		
If not Stage III or IV and patient is young and treatment would change if disease found, do surgical staging 1. Peritoneoscopy–Liver biopsy 2. Laparotomy–Liver biopsy, splenectomy, node biopsy	→	If positive for lymphoma, treat as advanced disease
↓		
If still no lymphoma is found, treat with local therapy.		

side of the diaphragm opposite that of the initial biopsy. Generally this will mean evaluation of the intraperitoneal and retroperitoneal structures. Depending on the patient's age and condition and the quality of the various studies performed at the institution, this will mean performing lymphangiography, abdominal CAT scan, or ultrasonography or a combination of these tests. If convincing evidence of lymphoma on the opposite side of the diaphragm is discovered, systemic therapy can generally be initiated. If the patient remains in Stage I or II after these studies *and* the patient is young *and* therapy would change if the findings were positive *and* the initial biopsy was above the diaphragm, the patient should be offered a staging laparotomy.

This should be preceded when possible by peritoneoscopy and liver biopsy which might obviate the need for the laparotomy. If the above criteria for performing a staging laparotomy are not met and the patient still has localized disease after nonsurgical staging, it is probably best to initiate local radiotherapy and reserve systemic therapy for those patients that recur.

Selected Reading

Best, J.J.K., Blackledge, G., Forbes, W.S.C., et al.: Computed tomography of abdomen in staging and clinical management of lymphoma. *Br. Med. J.* 2:1675–1677, 1978.

Carbone, P.P., Kaplan, H.S., Musshoff, K., et al.: Report of the Committee on Hodgkin's disease staging classification. *Cancer Res.* 31:1860–1861, 1971.

Castellino, R.A.: Lymphographic-histologic correlation in patients with Hodgkin's disease and non-Hodgkin's lymphoma undergoing staging laparotomy. *Lymphology* 7:153–157, 1974.

Castellino, R.A., Marglin, S.I., Carroll, B.A., et al.: The radiologic evaluation of abdominal and pelvic lymph nodes in oncologic practice. *Cancer Treatment Rev.* 7:153–160, 1980.

Chabner, B.A., Johnson, D.E., Young, R.C., et al.: Sequential nonsurgical and surgical staging of non-Hodgkin's lymphomas. *Ann. Intern. Med.* 85:149–154, 1976.

DeVita, V.T., Hellman, S.: Hodgkin's disease and the non-Hodgkin's lymphomas, in DeVita, V.T., Hellman, S., Rosenberg, S.A. (eds.): *Cancer: Principles and Practice of Oncology*. Philadelphia, J.B. Lippincott Co., 1982, pp. 1331–1401.

Horn, N.L., Ray, G.R., Kriss, J.P.: Gallium-67 citrate scanning in Hodgkin's disease and non-Hodgkin's lymphoma. *Cancer* 37:250–257, 1976.

Kaplan, H.S. (ed.): *Hodgkin's Disease*. Cambridge, Mass., Harvard Univ. Press, 1980.

Schechter, J.P., Jones, S.E., Woolfenden, J.M., et al.: Bone scanning in lymphoma. *Cancer* 38:1142–1148, 1976.

4

Surgical Aspects of Lymphoma

John G. Allison, M.D.

Introduction

Advances in the management and improvement in survival of most solid malignant neoplasms is frustratingly slow, but within the field of cancer therapy the most encouraging progress has been made in the lymphomas, and particularly so in Hodgkin's disease. Predicted survival rates have improved dramatically over the past 25 years in this subgroup. Better histopathological classification has identified subtypes in the non-Hodgkin's lymphomas which are more responsive to the therapeutic modalities available. The relatively orderly pathological advance of Hodgkin's disease, in contrast with the non-Hodgkin's lymphomas, has made accurate staging of the former a crucial factor in selecting appropriate therapy and planning adequate fields of radiation therapy. A cautiously optimistic attitude that Hodgkin's disease is eminently curable has been adopted, but this curability is dependent on adequate treatment of all known disease, either by irradiation to involved nodal regions or by systemic chemotherapy for disseminated disease. The radiotherapist and hematologist-oncologist are most closely involved with the management of the lymphoma patient, but the surgeon can contribute in a meaningful and positive way in both nodal and extranodal disease of all histological types.

This chapter will deal primarily with the role of surgery in the diagnosis, therapy, staging, and posttreatment restaging in Hodgkin's disease and non-Hodgkin's lymphoma (NHL). Although other chapters address the pathology, classification, and staging of Hodgkin's disease and NHL, for the sake of continuity there will be some repetition within the following paragraphs. The older pathological labels are compared with some of the newer ones in Table 1.

Table 1
Classification of Lymphomas

Hodgkin's Group	*Histological Type*	*Old Nomenclature*
Hodgkin's Disease	Lymphocyte Predominant	Paragranuloma
	Nodular Sclerosing	Granuloma
	Mixed Cell	—
	Lymphocyte Depleted	Sarcoma
Non-Hodgkin's Group	*Growth Pattern*	*Old Nomenclature*
Lymphocytic		
Well-Differentiated		Lymphosarcoma
Poorly Differentiated	Diffuse or Nodular	Giant Follicular Lymphoma
Histiocytic	Diffuse or Nodular	Reticulum Cell Sarcoma Giant Follicular Lymphoma
Mixed-Cell		
Histiocytic and Lymphocytic	Nodular	Giant Follicular Lymphoma

The multinucleated Reed-Sternberg giant cell is the diagnostic *sine qua non* of Hodgkin's disease, with subtyping based on the ratio of other cell types. With the exception of the nodular sclerosing subtype, the growth pattern tends to be diffuse. The precursor of the Reed-Sternberg cell remains controversial but evidence for its origin from a monocyte-macrophage has been reviewed recently by Kaplan. The histological types "lymphocyte predominant" and "nodular sclerosing" are generally regarded as "favorable histology" and carry a better long-term prognosis than either the "mixed cellular" or "lymphocyte-depleted" types.

Distinction between Hodgkin's disease and NHL and the latter's subtypes, based on cell types, cell size, and growth pattern (see Chapter 1) is critical to the further evaluation and subsequent treatment, and hence prognosis. Accurate staging in Hodgkin's disease would appear to have greater importance in determining treatment and prognosis than in NHL, although there are subtypes in the latter group in which such requirements may yet have therapeutic and prognostic implications.

Although there may be exceptions with some of the subtypes of NHL, the most widely used staging classification is that established in Ann Arbor, Michigan, in 1971. Four stages are identified.

Stage I: Involvement of a single lymph node region (Hodgkin's disease or NHL). A single extralymphatic organ or site (NHL only).

Stage II: Involvement of two or more noncontiguous lymph node regions on the same side of the diaphragm (Hodgkin's disease or NHL). Localized involvement of an extralymphatic organ and one or more lymph node groups on the same side of the diaphragm (NHL only).

Stage III: Involvement of lymph node regions on both sides of the diaphragm, which may or may not be associated with splenic involvement, or localized involvement of an extralymphatic organ, or both (Hodgkin's disease and NHL).

Stage IV: Diffuse or disseminated involvement of one or more extralymphatic organs, with or without associated lymph node involvement (Hodgkin's disease and NHL).

Extranodal organ involvement, proved on biopsy, may be designated by a suffix, e.g., Stage II-E. This would imply direct spread by contiguity from a node or nodes to an adjacent organ. Stage IV may be better defined by designating H^+ (liver involvement), M^+ (marrow involvement), and so forth. Further substaging into A or B is based on the presence or absence of systemic systems (fever, night sweats, and an unexplained 10% loss of weight in the preceding 6 months), which have been discussed in Chapter 3.

The precise roles of radiation therapy and chemotherapy have been addressed elsewhere in this text, but it is fairly widely accepted that the treatment of Hodgkin's disease in Stages I (A and B), II (A and B), and III (A) is radiotherapy. Multiagent chemotherapy is conventionally reserved as salvage treatment for relapses, but there is evidence that, when combined with irradiation, it may be of benefit in Stage III-A. Hodgkin's disease in Stages III-B and IV and the non-Hodgkin's lymphomas in all stages are usually treated by combination chemotherapy, with irradiation being reserved for local management of extranodal disease and rapid control of symptomatic bulky nodes.

Biopsy

Referral for biopsy of a suspicious lymph node or group of nodes, commonly in the neck, usually heralds the entry of the patient into the surgeon's sphere. Because of the influence of accurate histopathological diagnosis on therapy and prognosis, the quality of the biopsy material is of great concern to the pathologist. An intact whole node is preferred, and to achieve this a rather more generous incision than sometimes appears necessary may be required. It is not always necessarily the first node encountered that will yield diagnostic information and the largest and firmest node in that group, especially if there appears to be a surrounding reaction or adherence to adjacent structures, is more likely to prove fruitful. Most surgeons, at one time or another, have been confronted with a node that is deeper than at first appreciated by a palpation, or more difficult that anticipated to extirpate without mutilation. For this reason, although the majority of lymph node biopsies can be done with infiltration of local anesthetic, consideration should be given to the use of general anesthesia, either by choice or as "stand-by," when nodes are situated deep within the axilla or supraclavicular fossa. This pertains especially to children in whom the discomfort may produce restlessness leading to a troublesome dissection or break in sterile technique.

Meticulous dissection and hemostasis are essential. Traction on a node is best applied by using transfixion sutures (Fig. 1) rather than application of mutilating clamps. Smaller nodes may easily be encompassed in the jaws of a Babcock bowel forceps. Distortion of nodal architecture leads to diagnostic dilemmas, and the fresh node should be handed directly to the pathologist for fresh imprints ("touch preps") and subsequent fixation. A frozen section examination is helpful in establishing the diagnostic value of the nodes harvested. If no pathologist is available, several cross-sectional slices should be made in the node before fixation in formaldehyde. Failure to do so leads to poor permeation of the fixative and autolysis resulting in an inconclusive diagnosis and the need for a second biopsy.

Margolis and Organ reviewed 100 peripheral lymph node biopsies and discovered a disappointing diagnostic yield of only 48%. By attention to improvement in technique and an emphasis on delivering a whole intact node to the pathologist, they were able to increase their yield to 63% of a further 267 lymph nodes biopsied. When lymphoma was clinically suspected, a positive yield of 73% was achieved, although one-sixth of those in this group proved to have a disease other than lymphoma. The increasing use of electronmicroscopy in subtyping Hodgkin's disease and NHL requires a portion of the tissue, nodal or otherwise, to be fixed in glutaraldehyde rather than formaldehyde. A small fragment of fresh tissue should be placed on a saline-soaked gauze square, or in a balanced electrolyte tissue culture medium (not in saline), and handed to the immunopathologist within 15 to 20 minutes for the identification of immunological markers.

Biopsy of a soft-tissue mass in the patient with known or suspected lymphoma is occasionally required. All the principles outlined above apply and as much of the tumor as can be removed safely should be excised. A laparotomy for excisional biopsy of an intestinal tumor

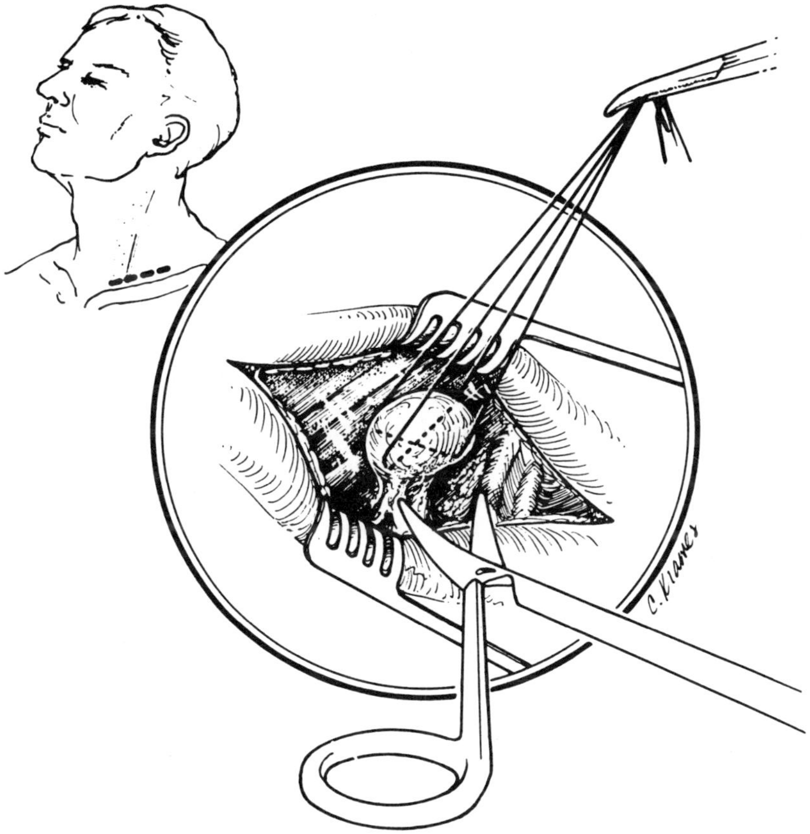

Figure 1: Biopsy of a left supraclavicular lymph node. The technique of transfixion sutures for retraction of a node to prevent distortion of nodal architecture is illustrated.

is required infrequently, but frozen section confirmation of the diagnosis is imperative as this may determine a need for a wide resection and the extent thereof. Incidental discovery of a suspicious lesion during the course of an abdominal operation for other reasons should be managed appropriately in order to obviate the potential for reexploration. Frozen section confirmation of a diagnosis of lymphoma is desirable. Once this has been made, the surgeon must then consider the merits of proceeding with a wide resection, or even to a formal staging procedure. Consultation with a hematologist-oncologist colleague before the abdomen is closed, to discuss the possible therapeutic options based on extent of disease and provisional histology, would be wise. Additional procedures, including staging by splenectomy and multiple node biopsies, would be acceptable when laparotomy has been done for an elective operation, such as cholecystectomy, but is definitely contraindicated and to be deprecated as an encore to emergency surgery or when an infectious process has been encountered within the peritoneal cavity.

Percutaneous needle liver biopsies and bone marrow biopsies, although minor surgical procedures, are usually done by the hematologist-oncologist during the course of the diagnostic and staging evaluation. The place for peritoneoscopy will be discussed in the section dealing with staging laparotomy.

Staging Laparotomy

No sooner had the impact of accurate staging on therapeutic and prognostic considerations been appreciated than the clinical evaluation in the pretreatment phase of patients with Hodgkin's disease and NHL was intensified. Fifty-five articles from the English literature, encompassing nearly 4,000 patients, have been reviewed and the results are summarized in Tables 2 and 3. This collected series includes patients with Hodgkin's disease and NHL and may help to reinforce some of the concepts expressed by Dr. Armitage in Chapter 3, *Evaluating the Patient with Lymphoma*, as well as clarify some of the cloudy issues surrounding the use and abuse of staging laparotomy.

The introduction of bipedal lymphangiography (LAG) into the diagnostic armamentarium greatly enhanced the detection of nodal disease below the diaphragm, but its accuracy varies considerably. The overall accuracy of LAG in Hodgkin's disease and NHL is 82% and 80% respectively, with a wide range and standard deviation, no doubt functions of the experience and expertise of those performing the procedure, as well as of the diligence of the surgeon in harvesting intraabdominal lymph nodes at staging laparotomy. The LAG false-negative rate in Hodgkin's disease ranges from 0% to 42% (mean 16.2%) and from 3% to 40% (mean 13.3%) in NHL. False-positive rates in both Hodgkin's disease and NHL are disturbingly high with a range of 8% to 90% (mean 34.7%) in the former and 4% to 80% (mean 29%) in the latter. This means that there are a significant number of patients, particularly those with Hodgkin's disease, in whom the disease is less likely to be widely disseminated at the time of diagnosis, who could be subjected to unnecessary aggressive therapy. The other side of the coin, however, is that some patients may be undertreated

Table 2
Data from 45 Reports* (3,081 Patients) on Staging Laparotomy for Hodgkin's Disease

	Number of Patients	Determinate Patients	Percent	Determinate Reports
Overall Stage Change	887	2,572	29%	41
Patients Up-staged**	454	2,054	22% (range 2–49)	28
Patients Down-staged	231	2,054	11% (range 0–62)	28
L.A.G.*** Accuracy			82 ± 8% (range 72–93)	9
L.A.G. False Positive			34.7 ± 21% (range 8–90)	20
L.A.G. False Negative			16.7 ± 14% (range 0–42)	20
Morbidity	225	1,800	14%	27
Mortality	8	2,559	0.3%	39

*Not all reports addressed the parameters in the table, hence the discrepancy in numbers of "determinate" data.
**Upstaging refers to advancing the stage, i.e., more extensive disease discovered on laparotomy.
***L.A.G. = bipedal lymphangiography.

and denied the possibility of cure if decisions on therapy are based on the results of LAG alone. There exists, also, a gray zone in which the lymphangiograms are interpreted as "equivocal"; the majority of these prove to be negative after histological examination of the nodes. Lymphangiography will, of course, demonstrate only those nodal groups in continuity and is unable to provide information about the mesenteric, porta hepatis, celiac axis, and splenic hilar nodes. Filling and interpretation of the upper abdominal periaortic nodes is often inadequate and thus even less reliable. This may have some implications, depending on the therapeutic policies of an individual institution, on the management of patients with Hodgkin's disease where treatment of Stage III_1 (nodal disease above the transverse mesocolon) is different from treatment of Stage III_2 (nodal disease below the transverse mesocolon).

Table 3
Data from 10 Reports* (834 Patients) on Staging Laparotomy for Non-Hodgkin's Lymphoma

	Number of Patients	Determinate Patients	Percent	Determinate Reports
Overall Stage Change	333	765	44%	9
Patients Up-staged***	312	765	41% (range 23–84)	9
Patients Down-staged	21	765	3% (range 0–13)	9
L.A.G.*** Accuracy			80 ± 23% (range 45–96)	4
L.A.G. False Positive			29 ± 34% (range 4–80)	4
L.A.G. False Negative			13 ± 18% (range 3–40)	

*Not all reports addressed the parameters in the table, hence the discrepancy in numbers of "determinate" data.
**Upstaging refers to advancing the stage, i.e., more extensive disease discovered on laparotomy.
***L.A.G. = bipedal lymphangiography.

The introduction by Glatstein et al., in 1969, of pretreatment laparotomy as part of the staging protocol in lymphoma heralded a major advance in the management and prognosis, particularly of Hodgkin's disease. Wide application of this diagnostic tool since then has demonstrated that clinical staging into Stages I, II, and III is incorrect in almost one-third of cases. The collected review reveals that 887 of 2,572 determinant patients with Hodgkin's disease (29%) had their clinical stage changed following laparotomy. There were 454 of 2,054 determinant patients (22%) who had their disease upstaged, i.e., more extensive disease was discovered, with a range of 2% to 49% within the series. Two hundred and thirty-one of these 2,054 patients (11%) were downstaged, i.e., the disease was less extensive than previously believed, with a range of 0% to 62% within the series. In those studies examining the effect of staging laparotomy on stage change in NHL, there were only 21 of 765 determinant patients (3%) who were downstaged. Three hundred and twelve of these 765 (41%)

were upstaged, with an overall change of stage in 44%. A difference within the NHL subtype, particularly with regard to growth pattern, on the stage alteration was observed. Fewer than 10% of patients with nodular NHL will have their stage changed, while as many as 30% of those classified as diffuse (most of them of the histiocytic subtype) will undergo a revision of their stage. This may have some marginal value in assessing prognosis, but it is to be emphasized that unless an alteration of stage results in alteration in therapy, these data for NHL are quite meaningless. Although 44% had a stage change, this led to a change in the therapeutic approach in very few cases.

Detection of intraabdominal nodal disease not revealed by LAG, and of splenic involvement not suspected clinically, leads to the stage of disease being advanced and avails the patient of treatment that might otherwise have been denied. By the same token, patients who have their clinical stage reduced when laparotomy does not confirm the presence of subdiaphragmatic disease may be spared therapy not in fact required. Errors in lymphangiographic interpretation are disclosed and nonvisualized nodal groups may be sampled.

There is a consensus that there exists little correlation between preoperative, or even intraoperative, assessment of the spleen and the finite histological diagnosis in Hodgkin's disease. As many as 61% of spleens palpable before operation and considered to be harboring Hodgkin's disease will prove to be histologically negative, while 21% to 38% of those regarded as innnocent by clinical assessment will return a positive histology. Mitchell and Peters reported an overall 43% inaccuracy in preoperative splenic scans—38% false-negative and 47% false-positive. There is a better correlation in NHL with nearly two-thirds of palpable spleens being involved. Whereas the weight of the spleen matters little as far as the final histological evaluation is concerned in Hodgkin's disease, more than 50% of spleens weighing 200 grams or more in NHL will be positive, as will 100% weighing more than 400 grams.

Liver involvement by either Hodgkin's disease or NHL may be detected by percutaneous liver biopsy. This is especially indicated when there are disturbances in serological liver function tests (of which an elevated alkaline phosphatase is the most sensitive) or an abnormal liver scan. A positive biopsy result automatically places the patient in Stage IV (assuming nodal disease proved elsewhere), but a negative biopsy result does not exclude hepatic involvement. Furthermore, there may be liver involvement without elevation of liver enzymes or bilirubin, and in the face of a normal liver scan. Open liver biopsy is far more sensitive and may well reverse the findings of a negative needle biopsy. As there are no afferent lymphatics to the spleen, it is believed that the most common method of spread to the subdiaphragmatic area in Hodgkin's disease is via hematogenous routes to the spleen. This concept, and the belief that Hodgkin's disease does indeed spread by continuity through the lymphatic system, is supported by the fact that the splenic hilar, suprapancreatic, and celiac axis nodes are the earliest to be involved in subdiaphragmatic disease (remember that these nodal groups cannot be visualized on LAG). In only 3% of cases where hepatic involvement with Hodgkin's disease has been histologically confirmed will the spleen be free of disease. When the spleen is involved, however, the liver will be involved in 45% of cases.

The impact of changing the stage, especially in Hodgkin's disease, based on the findings at laparotomy is primarily on the treatment; the extent of the field to be irradiated may be altered or the use of combination chemotherapy rather than radiotherapy indicated. The place and extent of radiation therapy for Hodgkin's disease is discussed more extensively in Chapter 7, but by and large the treatment of choice for disease confined above the diaphragm (Stages I and II, A or B) is a mantle field of irradiation. Stage III-A, however, is best treated by nodal irradiation that incorporates the mantle above with an inverted Y-shaped field below the diaphragm, or even by total nodal irradiation. Splenectomy at the time of staging laparotomy obviates the need to include the left upper quadrant in the area to be irradiated, thus reducing the risk of radiation pneumonitis or nephritis. Reducing the stage from IV to III or even from III to II protects the patient against unnecessary overtreatment. The risk of leukemia which has been reported as occurring in some who have combined modality treatment can thereby be reduced. Conversely, those who have their stage advanced to III-A can be offered the extended field of irradiation required to treat the disease adequately. Advancing the stage to III-B or IV would, in most centers, mandate combination chemotherapy. A randomized study, which contrasted patients (in clinical Stages I or II-A) whose staging included a laparotomy with those staged without laparotomy, showed an abdominal relapse rate of 5% in the former group and 31% in the latter, highlighting the value of the procedure in identifying those in whom more extensive treatment is warranted.

Much controversy surrounds the use of staging laparotomy, especially in Hodgkin's disease, and its appropriateness depends to a certain extent on the institution in which the patient is being treated. There are, for example, some who believe that Stage II Hodgkin's disease, and perhaps even Stage I, especially if the B symptoms are present, should be treated by an extended mantle field of irradiation. This extends caudad to incorporate the intraabdominal periaortic nodes and the spleen but does not extend below the bifurcation of the aorta. It is axiomatic that the benefits of such an extended port be greater than the risks of unnecessary irradiation of bowel, vertebrae, and other intraabdominal organs, when weighed against the benefits and risks of staging laparotomy which has the potential for obviating such an extended port.

Pretreatment staging laparotomy may not be indicated in a select subpopulation of patients with Hodgkin's disease because of the extremely low incidence of upstaging the disease when certain criteria are met. These criteria would include young females with clinical Stage I disease, favorable histology (i.e., nodular sclerosing or lymphocyte predominant), and a negative LAG. B symptoms should be absent. As the thoracic duct usually drains into the left subclavian vein, and current understanding of Hodgkin's disease predicts its spread by lymphatic continuity, primary nodal disease in the right axilla or supraclavicular fossa is less likely to be associated with subdiaphragmatic disease than when the diagnosis is made following biopsy of nodes on the left side. Because the positive yield of staging laparotomy in this group is low, it has been suggested that surgical exploration of the abdomen be withheld because of the mortality and morbidity of the procedure. One must nevertheless bear in mind that there will be certain persons denied the advantage of adequate treatment. The application of statistics to the individual carries an inherent danger that eminently curable disease may be left untreated. The question is a contentious one but the problem may have been resolved by the introduction of restaging, or posttreatment, laparotomy (*vide infra*). Subdiaphragmatic relapse is more common with the mixed cellularity or lymphocyte-depleted subtypes of Hodgkin's disease and the use of extended field radiotherapy without staging laparotomy for those may well be appropriate for all stages other than III-B and IV.

The importance of relating the need for staging laparotomy in Hodgkin's disease to the radiotherapeutic policies of any given institution is pointed out very neatly by Dent and his colleagues in their review of 100 cases undergoing staging laparotomy in Cape Town, South Africa (Table 4). Of these patients, 28 had their stage changed. By applying three hypothetical radiotherapeutic programs to all 100 patients, it becomes apparent that 72 would have been excessively treated had they received total nodal irradiation, but that none would have disease left untreated. In a program where total nodal or extended field irradiation, selected according to stage, would be used, eight

Table 4
Appropriateness or Otherwise of Three Hypothetical Radiotherapeutic Programs

	Irradiation		
	Total Nodal	Extended Field	Mantle
Radical Program I	(N = 100)		
Appropriate	28		
Excessive	72		
Missed disease	0		
Radical Program II	(N = 13)	(N = 87)	
Appropriate	5+	22	
Excessive	8	64	
Missed disease	0	1	
Conservative Program	(N = 13)	(N = 39)	(N = 48)
Appropriate	5+	11	36
Excessive	8	28*	0
Missed disease	0	0	12

*These 28 patients had mediastinal disease and extended-field therapy would have been appropriate to the protocol.
+Five patients with apparent stage IIIB disease would have received chemotherapy; 2 of these were restaged as IIB after laparotomy.
Reproduced from Dent, et al., *South African Medical Journal* 62:509–511, 1982, with permission of the publishers.

would have received excessive treatment had they undergone total nodal irradiation and 64 with the extended field. One patient in the latter group would have been undertreated. When the extent of irradiation includes total nodal, extended field, and mantle field, again selected on stage decided without laparotomy, eight would have received unnecessary total nodal irradiation, but 12 patients undergoing mantle field irradiation would have been undertreated.

Another hotly debated issue is the place for splenectomy as part of a staging procedure, especially in children younger than 10 years. The syndrome of overwhelming postsplenectomy infection has been well documented. It is seen most frequently in asplenic children and is believed to be related to an impairment of an immunological response to the capsular antigen of certain bacteria, notably the *Hemophilus* strains and *Streptococcus pneumoniae*. The syndrome is seen sporadically in adults and it is likely that previous exposure to these organisms, with better antigenic recognition, provides protection.

Because of a *de facto* immunological deficiency in Hodgkin's disease, it is open to speculation whether splenectomy in these children does increase the risk of sepsis, particularly in those cases in which the spleen is already involved. For the reasons that staging laparotomy results in a stage change more frequently in children than in adults

(35% to 50%) and LAG is more difficult to perform and more difficult to interpret, staging laparotomy has the potential for a greater impact on altering the therapeutic approach. The incidence of postsplenectomy infection in reports which specifically address this question range from 0% to 5%. The true meaning of this has been challenged as surveys have shown that no difference may exist between splenectomized children and those who develop overwhelming sepsis when no splenectomy has been performed. The ravages of the underlying disease and immunological suppression by irradiation therapy or combination chemotherapy are unquestionably factors in such a catastrophic event, even when the spleen has been preserved. Furthermore, the frequency of overwhelming postsplenectomy infection appears to be lower in those who have had their spleens removed as part of a staging procedure than in those who have undergone splenectomy for other reasons (e.g., trauma). It appears, too, that splenectomized children with Hodgkin's disease may tolerate radiotherapy and chemotherapy better. It has been suggested that partial splenectomy for staging may suffice, but this has been countered by the argument that 11.5% of patients reported by Dearth et al. had the only site of their abdominal Hodgkin's disease limited to a few nodules in a localized distribution and without visible subcapsular lesions—these would have gone undetected by partial splenectomy. The patients would therefore have been understaged and inadequately treated. The devastating effects of irradiation on vertebral maturation and spinal growth and the incidence of induced second malignant neoplasms are worrisome, but the value and curative potential of radiotherapy in Hodgkin's disease mitigate against its hazards. An alternative that has been suggested to avoid these complications of radiation therapy is to treat Hodgkin's disease in all young children under 10 years with chemotherapy *ab initio*. Neither laparotomy nor splenectomy would then be indicated for primary staging.

If the decision to proceed with formal staging laparotomy, including splenectomy, is made in children, administration of prophylactic penicillin by mouth for several years afterwards, with or without the use of vaccines currently available, would be a wise precaution.

Initial enthusiasm for peritoneoscopically directed biopsy of liver or spleen, or both, has waned. Liver biopsy specimens are perforce small and the sensitivity is not much greater than that of percutaneous needle biopsy. Its value in evaluating splenic involvement is limited for the same reasons mentioned earlier. (Many surgeons, also, would shudder at the thought of biting a hole in the spleen without having immediate recourse to a means of controlling the possible ensuing hemorrhage!)

In summary, it can be said that staging laparotomy still has an important role to play in the management of selected patients with Hodgkin's disease and as a scientific tool within strictly controlled protocols designed to further the understanding of the natural history and behavior following treatment. In those institutions where there is a spectrum of treatment, the policies being decided on strict staging, the recommendation for more or less aggressive radiation therapy, or for systemic chemotherapy, may be influenced. The procedure is then most certainly indicated. Its application in institutions where a more aggressive policy of radiation therapy has been adopted, particularly for the lower stages, will obviously be more limited. Its thoughtless use is to be deplored, for scientific and ethical reasons.

Routine laparotomy for the staging of NHL can no longer be justified. It does have a role in circumstances where, for example, a histiocytic lymphoma has been diagnosed in an extranodal site and conventional investigations failed to disclose nodal or other extranodal disease. NHL exhibiting a nodular growth pattern is invariably widespread at the time of diagnosis and combination chemotherapy is usually recommended *per primam*. Demonstration of intraabdominal disease would not radically alter the treatment policy. The incidence of downstaging NHL through staging laparotomy is only 3%, although some have reported a rate as high as 30% when the growth pattern is of the diffuse type. The histiocytic lymphoma, when confined to a local area, is amenable to local field irradiation, with or without a preceding debulking surgical procedure, and when this is suspected, a staging laparotomy to exclude disseminated disease may well be indicated. As the yield in terms of modifying treatment through alteration of the clinical stage is low in NHL, routine staging laparotomy has been abandoned. The results of a combined series of reports reviewing staging laparotomy in NHL is summarized in Table 3.

Staging Laparotomy: The Operation

Although there exists a definite place for staging laparotomy in the management of Hodgkin's disease and occasionally in NHL, its success and value are predicated by the quality of the operation. To subject a patient to a major abdominal operation and have subdiaphragmatic disease missed because of an inadequate procedure is rather self-defeating. The technique of primary staging laparotomy is well established and has been extensively discussed in the literature. For the operation to maintain its rightful place in the management of lymphoma, strict attention to technique should be maintained to provide maximum information, and thus benefit, to the patient.

A transverse or chevron incision has been described, but a midline incision extending from the xiphoid to well below the umbilicus is preferred. The first procedure performed on gaining access to the peritoneal cavity should be the liver biopsy. Artifactual changes in the liver with distortion of architecture and a round cell infiltrate resulting from prolonged and often over-enthusiastic retraction may, under certain circumstances, lead to some confusion in the pathologist's interpretation of the histological features. Although of less importance in Hodgkin's disease, it may be critical on those rare occasions when a staging laparotomy is being done for NHL. Nuclear distortion of cells in an infiltrate may be confused with the cleft nuclei, one of the distinguishing histological features used in subtyping the lymphocytic lymphomas.

Substantial wedge biopsy specimens from the anterior edges of both right and left lobes of the liver should be taken. Hemostasis is best secured by deeply placed compression sutures of heavy chromic catgut, taking a single wide bite with each and snugging down the knots on the outer surface. This permits Glisson's capsule to buttress the suture and prevent tearing of the liver substance (Fig. 2). No

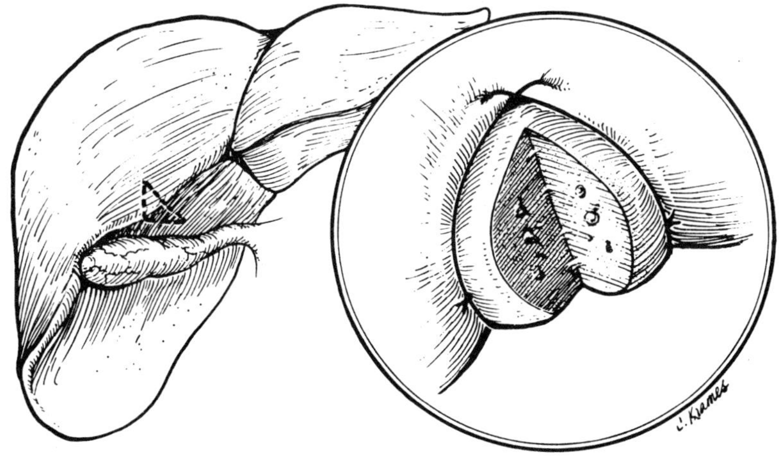

Figure 2: A wedge biopsy from the anterior edge of the right lobe of the liver. The technique of compression sutures for hemostasis is depicted in the inset. A similar wedge biopsy should be taken from the left lobe.

attempt should be made to approximate the cut edges by tying together the free ends of these sutures. Application of diathermy may be necessary to control small bleeding points and, as a precautionary measure, vessels or biliary radicals large enough to be identified with the naked eye should be ligated or suture-ligated with fine silk. At least two deep needle biopsies (Tru-cut) should then be taken, one from each lobe, although more are preferred. The biopsy needles should be directed away from the hilum of the liver to lessen the chance of puncturing a major bile duct or large vessel. Oozing from the puncture site can be controlled by pressure applied to the liver surface for three to four minutes. Any suspicious nodule on the surface or mass within the parenchyma of the liver should be biopsied first and submitted for frozen section. If this is positive, no further liver biopsy need be done.

A comprehensive exploration of the abdominal cavity, including inspection and palpation of the liver, spleen, stomach, pancreas, and the whole bowel, should not be omitted. The retroperitoneal space, particularly the renal fossae, should be palpated for any abnormality in renal contour or retroperitoneal masses. Any suspicious lesions should be biopsied and submitted for frozen section.

Careful and conscientious sampling of all lymph node groups is mandatory. The preaortic and periaortic lymph nodes are exposed by reflecting the transverse colon cephalad and retracting the small bowel to the right. Use of a Lahey bag helps facilitate this maneuver and may reduce the incidence of postoperative adhesions. The peritoneum is opened alongside the aorta from its bifurcation to the duodenum and left renal vein. Nodes on the anterior surface of the aorta and lying between it and the inferior mesenteric vein and left ureter are exposed by a combination of careful sharp and blunt dissection (Fig. 3). Lymphangiographic abnormalities of the iliac nodes on either side, or the therapeutic policies of that particular institution, may require that these groups of nodes be sampled too. Having the preoperative lymphangiogram in the operating room may be helpful in identifying those nodes most likely to be positive. Intraoperative roentgenograms will confirm that these have been removed. Hemostasis is secured and the peritoneal incision over the aorta closed with a running suture of absorbable material.

The small bowel and colon are then returned to their anatomical positions and attention directed to the upper abdomen. The lesser sac should be entered by opening the gastrocolic ligament, extending this up to the cardia of the stomach by dividing and ligating the short gastric vessels. Care should be exercised not to include a portion of

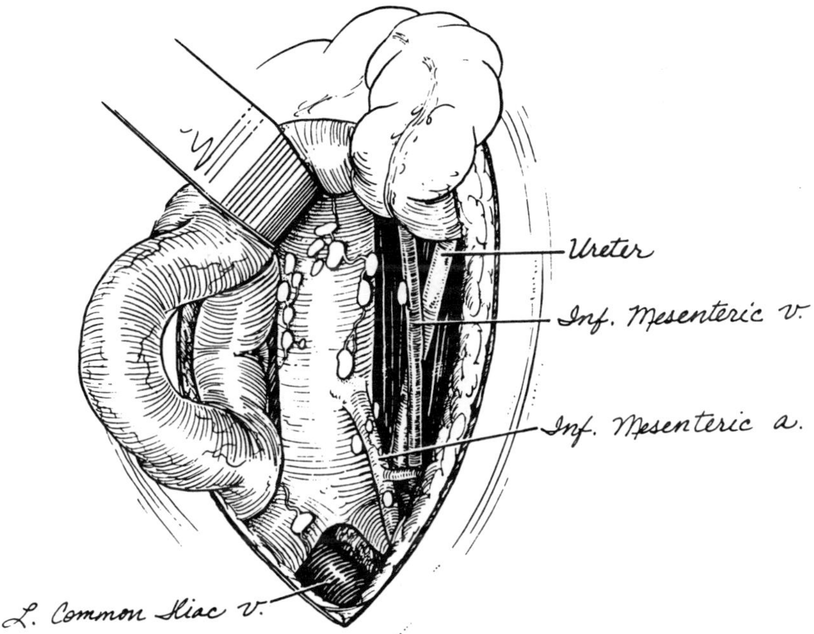

Figure 3: Exposure of the abdominal aorta and retroperitoneal structures after incision of the posterior peritoneum. The transverse colon and small bowel have been retracted and the aorta exposed from its bifurcation to the left renal vein (hidden). Exposure of the bifurcations of both common iliac arteries may be necessary in some circumstances. Several nodes should be sampled, especially larger ones and those that are believed to correspond to abnormal nodes detected on bipedal lymphangiography.

the stomach wall in the ligated pedicles as this may be complicated by local necrosis and gastric perforation. Having opened the lesser sac, the suprapancreatic nodes can be sampled, after which the spleen is mobilized by dividing the lienophrenic and lienocolic ligaments. The splenic artery and vein may be divided anteriorly near the tail of the pancreas (transfixion sutures are recommended for these vesssels) or they may be taken from behind after rotation of the spleen and tail of the pancreas into the incision. Damage to the tail of the pancreas should be avoided. The splenic bed is packed with laparotomy pads and the celiac axis group of nodes exposed by opening the gastrohepatic ligament and retracting the intraabdominal esophagus and gastric cardia to the left (Fig. 4). This maneuver is facilitated by complete exposure of the lesser sac after the greater curve of the stomach has been mobilized prior to splenectomy. It is imperative that biopsies are

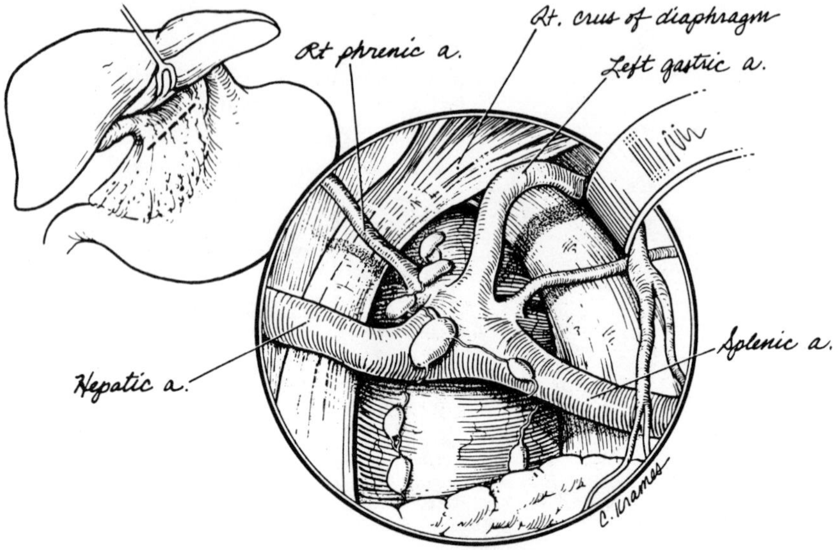

Figure 4: Exposure of the celiac axis following incision of the gastrohepatic ligament is achieved by retracting the lesser curve of the stomach, together with the descending branch of the left gastric artery and intraabdominal esophagus to the left.

performed on these groups of nodes (splenic hilar, suprapancreatic, and celiac axis) in Hodgkin's disease as they are the earliest to be involved. Nodes in the porta hepatis and pyloric region are exposed by kocherizing the duodenum and incising the peritoneum anterior to the common bile duct. Prominent nodes that may easily be identified are those of the cystic duct and distal common bile duct.

Suspicious nodes in the mesenteries of the small bowel and transverse sigmoid colon should then be looked for. These are seldom involved in Hodgkin's disease but are not uncommon sites in which NHL may be detected.

A tantalum clip should be placed at the site of every node biopsy and the splenic pedicle similarly marked by a small cluster of clips, preferably of a different size. The use of clips for purposes of hemostasis should be avoided as the result may be a roentgenographic "confusogram." Tantalum is preferred to stainless steel or silver. Visible on the roentgenogram, it does not produce the "starburst" artifact on the CAT scan and interfere with the interpretation of these at follow-up examinations.

If radiation policies include an inverted Y-field of irradiation, oophoropexy should be performed in female patients. Fixing the ovaries posterior to the uterus probably affords more protection than doing so to the lateral pelvic walls, as has been suggested by some. Fixation of the ovaries to the uterus can be accomplished by transfixing both with a single suture of monofilament polypropylene and including a healthy bit of myometrium. Because oophoropexy is associated with complications of amenorrhea, sterility, and dyspareunia, a recommendation has been made that the ovaries subsequently be relocated to their normal position. (It has not been reported but consideration might be given to peritoneoscopic or culdoscopic division of the fixation suture and relocation when irradiation has been completed and before adhesions become too dense.)

Other "encore" procedures may be appropriate. Appendectomy at the time of staging laparotomy is advised by some, the rationale being less from the detection of suspected disease but rather to avoid diagnostic dilemmas should the patient present at a later date with abdominal pain. Others have criticized this maneuver, primarily for fear of increasing the incidence of postoperative complications, but this should not occur in the face of sound surgical technique. Incidental appendectomy during hysterectomy or cholecystectomy has not been associated with an increased complication rate. If occult gallstones are discovered, the gallbladder should be removed, thus elminating the possible need for later cholecystectomy in a patient who has received a substantial dose of abdominal irradiation. Inclusion of the gallbladder in the preoperative ultrasonographic examination would seem to be a logical step to take in planning the laparotomy.

After adequate hemostasis has been secured, the abdomen is closed in the method of the surgeon's choice, although use of a nonabsorbable suture material is strongly recommended.

From the collected reviews mortality attributable directly to staging laparotomy is low. Eight deaths in 2,559 patients (0.3%) were recorded, although an isolated incidence of a 2% mortality rate has been reported. The procedure does carry the reputation of having a relatively high morbidity rate; complications in 225 of 1,800 patients (14%) were recorded in the reports reviewed.

An "unexplained postoperative fever" is common but without apparent sequelae. The more common serious complications encountered are wound infection, with a high rate of wound dehiscence, basal atelectasis, and urinary tract infection. Postoperative small bowel obstruction is not infrequent and usually follows adherence of a loop of bowel to the site of a node biopsy. Left subphrenic abscess, pancreatitis, and pancreatic fistula have also been reported. Iatrogenic complications resulting from damage to the ureter, hepatic artery, inferior vena cava, and colon have occurred but are avoidable.

Some controversy surrounds the incidence of deep vein thrombosis following splenectomy, and in particular splenectomy associated with staging laparotomy. As many as 50% of deep vein thromboses may be silent and remain clinically undetected; the reported incidence is therefore a function of the intensity for which it is sought. When routinely measured by the radioiodinated fibrinogen technique, the incidence after staging laparotomy is between 15% and 20%. Not all may be clinically significant and the incidence of postoperative pulmonary embolus after staging laparotomy appears to be no higher than that following other major surgery. One case of thrombotic thrombocytopenic purpura has been documented.

With a mortality rate of 0.3%, the rather high rate of postoperative morbidity should not serve to disparage the use and value of staging laparotomy in Hodgkin's disease, but should rather urge the surgeons concerned to strive for optimal preoperative preparation and meticulous attention to well-founded surgical principles.

Restaging Laparotomy in Hodgkin's Disease

The fairly recent introduction of posttreatment laparotomy in patients with Hodgkin's disease who have completed their course of radiotherapy or combination chemotherapy has identified some patients in whom residual untreated or partially treated disease remains. As the cure rate for Hodgkin's disease is closely allied to the 5-year remission rate, identification of such residual disease has cast doubt on the term "relapse" or "recurrence." The 5-year relapse rate of 5% for Stages I and II and 30% for Stage IV correlates very closely with the incidence of residual disease found below the diaphragm in patients undergoing posttreatment laparotomy. The detection of disease either not included in the radiation field, or incompletely treated as the result of inadequate radiation therapy or chemotherapy, warrants further treatment by either modality to eradicate the disease. Selection of these patients for further treatment should thus reduce the "relapse" rate and provide a greater chance for cure.

Posttreatment laparotomy is particularly relevant when persistent disease is suspected on the basis of clinical evaluation during follow-up. These have been addressed in an earlier chapter but would include an elevated sedimentation rate, rising serum copper levels, positive refill lymphangiography, isotope scanning, abdominal ultrasonography, or CAT scan. Unless suspicion of residual or recurrent disease is regarded as a criterion for further treatment, restaging by laparotomy is indicated. Even without the suggestion that further treatment may be required, untreated or partially treated disease may nevertheless be detected in patients considered to be in complete remission. The results of 49 patients studied by Sutcliffe et al. are summarized in Table 5. These patients had all completed a course of radiation therapy or combination chemotherapy; 61% of the former had either partially ablated or unchanged disease disclosed by laparotomy. Of these, seven had not had pretreatment laparotomy and were undergoing planned staging. Further treatment could be offered to those in whom disease was detected, the others being spared the distress of further therapy. Four of the 21 patients (19%) who had received combination chemotherapy were found to have persistent subdiaphragmatic disease. Four of the 19 patients in this group who were believed to be in complete remission required continued treatment, while two patients in whom residual disease was suspected were spared further treatment.

The benefits of restaging laparotomy have been shown by others. Coon et al. described 35 patients with Hodgkin's disease, of various stages, who had received either radiotherapy or combination chemotherapy. Secondary staging disclosed residual abdominal disease in 20. All 35 patients were suspected of harboring residual disease. Coker et al. performed 47 restaging laparotomies in 39 patients (six patients underwent two or more operations). Of these, 20 patients had undergone prior radiotherapy, 10 underwent chemotherapy and 9 underwent a combination of the two. Of these 47 laparotomies, 13 were

Table 5
Partially Ablated or Unmodified-Residual Abdominal Hodgkin's Disease at Posttreatment Laparotomy*

Radiotherapy (N = 28)		Chemotherapy (N = 21)	
Result	No.	Result	No.
Delayed Staging		In Remission	
Positive	3	Positive	4
Negative	4	Negative	15
Suspected-Residual HD		Suspected-Residual HD	
Positive	14	Positive	0
Negative	7	Negative	2

*From Sutcliffe et al., *Lancet* 2:57–60, 1978.

done for suspected residual Hodgkin's disease (after treatment had been completed) and four proved to be positive. Fifteen of 21 laparotomies done for clinically suspected relapse of intraabdominal disease were positive, following a median 36-month disease-free interval. Ten laparotomies were carried out on patients who presented with recurrence in a peripheral node and five of these disclosed intraabdominal Hodgkin's disease. Of three patients undergoing laparotomy to document complete response, one was found to have subdiaphragmatic nodal disease. The 22 patients who had negative restaging laparotomies all remained clinically free of disease for a median of 63 months.

Documentation of abdominal Hodgkin's disease by restaging laparotomy mandates further intensive therapy; failure to do so spares the patient from unnecessary treatment of a potentially harmful nature.

Although still under scrutiny and not unanimously accepted, the role of posttreatment, or restaging, laparotomy in patients with Hodgkin's disease, who have completed a course of radiotherapy or combination chemotherapy and in whom residual abdominal disease is suspected, seems justified. Its value and routine use, however, in patients considered to be in complete remission have yet to be established, although there is a small percentage of these patients who would obviously benefit by the procedure. Patients likely to fall into this category are those with the histological subtypes associated with mixed cellularity or lymphocyte depletion. There has been little experience with posttreatment laparotomy in NHL, but the available evidence suggests that it has no merit.

As with primary staging laparotomy, the use of restaging laparotomy, in the light of current knowledge, should either be confined to research protocols examining the natural history of the disease or be tailored to meet the investigational capabilities and therapeutic policies of the institution at which the patient is being treated.

Therapeutic Surgery in Lymphoma

Surgery in Hodgkin's disease and NHL is not limited to that for diagnosis or staging. The occasion may arise where excision or excisional biopsy of a large lymphomatous mass may have therapeutic advantages. Wide excision assists the oncologist or radiotherapist by reducing the tumor load and may, in cases where stomach or bowel is involved, obviate some of the complications that sometimes follow local irradiation or chemotherapy. The importance of the surgical management of lymphomas arising primarily in the gastrointestinal tract is dealt with in Chapter 5.

Stricture formation and intestinal obstruction at the site of a small bowel lymphoma require abdominal exploration with local resection, as may hemorrhage from a necrotic tumor mass. Free perforation into the peritoneal cavity is not uncommon, especially where there has been a rapid response of a transmural lymphomatous deposit to combination chemotherapy. Early appreciation of abdominal distention and free intraperitoneal air when this occurs will lead to prompt surgical intervention and the opportunity to perform resection and primary end-to-end anastomosis before a diffuse bacterial peritonitis supervenes.

Compression of adjacent organs by a bulky tumor may occasionally require surgical relief. Compression of the pyloroduodenal area by a retroperitoneal lymphoma, requiring temporary gastrostomy and feeding jejunostomy until response to local irradiation relieved the obstruction, has been reported. More critical is compression of the spinal cord or corda equina by lymphoma (usually extradural) resulting in a rapidly progressive paraparesis. Response to local irradiation may not be swift enough to prevent permanent neurological damage and loss of bladder and anorectal function. Urgent laminectomy is recommended in these circumstances. Mediastinal masses producing the superior vena cava syndrome, if not too far advanced, may be treated appropriately with irradiation, but a life-threatening situation or tardy response could well necessitate the urgent insertion of a spiral vein graft between one or other subclavian veins and the right atrium. Smaller lymphomatous masses of the breasts are adequately treated by local excision and irradiation, although consideration should be given to simple or modified radical mastectomy when the tumor is bulky or there is obvious axillary nodal involvement.

There are no strict guidelines governing when an operation is indicated, or even what procedure is appropriate, and the timing and selection of any operation depends on careful assessment of the patient and sound clinical judgment.

There is no doubt that the care of patients with lymphoma is multidisciplinary. The intricacies of the therapeutic and diagnostic requirements of lymphoma are so diverse that they are best handled by a panel of oncologists, radiotherapists, radiologists, pathologists, and surgeons. Interdisciplinary discussion and decision making can only benefit the individual patient, extend the knowledge and understanding of the disease and its behavior, and ultimately improve the prognosis. To have an interested surgeon participating in these discussions is preferable to having one involved only as a "mechanic" who harvests lymph nodes, surgically explores abdomens, and plucks spleens on a random referral basis. The surgeon needs to pay attention to the quality of tissue submitted to the pathologist and to the diligence with which the abdomen is explored in the search for previously undetected disease. Intact lymph nodes, biopsy specimens not macerated by careless handling, and well-planned laparotomies can only enhance diagnostic and staging accuracy. The most appropriate treatment may then be offered to the individual patient.

Selected Reading

Abrahamsen, A.F., Host, H., Jorgensen, O.G.: Is staging laparotomy of therapeutic value in patients with supradiaphragmatic Hodgkin's disease, clinical stage IA-IIA? *Scand. J. Hematol.* 25:439–444, 1980.

Botnick, L.E., Goodman, R., Jasse, N., et al.: Stages I-III Hodgkin's disease in children: Results of staging and treatment. *Cancer* 39:599–603, 1977.

Chabner, B.A., Johnson, R.E., Young, R.C., et al.: Sequential nonsurgical and surgical staging of non-Hodgkin's lymphoma. *Cancer* 42:922–925, 1978.

Cohen, I.T., Higgins, G.R., Powars, D.R., et al.: Staging laparotomy for Hodgkin's disease in children. *Arch. Surg.* 112:948–951, 1977.

Coker, D.B., Morris, D.M., Coleman, J.J., et al.: Restaging laparotomy for Hodgkin's disease. *Ann. Surg.* 197:79–83, 1983.

Coon, W.W., Dabich, L., Votaw, M.L.: "Secondary" operative staging of patients with lymphoma. *Arch. Surg.* 115:401–404, 1980.

Cooper, A., Ironside, P.N.J., Madigan, J.P., et al.: The role of splenectomy in the management of advanced Hodgkin's disease. *Cancer* 34:408–417, 1974.

Dearth, J.C., Gilchrist, G.S., Telander, R.L., et al.: Partial splenectomy for staging Hodgkin's disease: Risk of false-negative results. *N. Engl. J. Med.* 299:345–346, 1978.

Dent, D.M., King, H.S., Jacobs, P.: Is staging laparotomy necessary in Hodgkin's disease? *South African Med. J.* 62:509–511, 1982.

Givler, R.L., Brunk, S.F., Hass, C.A., et al.: Problems of interpretation of liver biopsy in Hodgkin's disease. *Cancer* 28:1335–1342, 1971.

Glatstein, E., Guernsey, J.M., Rosenberg, S.A., et al.: The value of laparotomy and splenectomy in the staging of Hodgkin's disease. *Cancer* 24:704–718, 1969.

Glees, J.P., Barr, L.C., McElwain, T.J., et al.: The changing role of staging laparotomy in Hodgkin's disease: A personal series of 310 patients. *Br. J. Surg.* 69:181–187, 1982.

Hancock, B.W., Bruce, L., Ward, A.M., et al.: Changes in immune status in patients undergoing splenectomy for the staging of Hodgkin's disease. *Br. Med. J.* 1:313–315, 1976.

Hays, E.M.: The staging of Hodgkin's disease in children reviewed. *Cancer* 35:973–978, 1975.

Hays, E.M., Karon, N., Isaacs, H., et al.: Hodgkin's disease: Technique and results of staging laparotomy in children. *Arch. Surg.* 106:507–512, 1973.

Ihde, D.C., DeVita, V.T., Canellos, G.P., et al.: Effect of splenectomy on tolerance to combination chemotherapy in patients with lymphoma. *Blood* 47:211–222, 1976.

Kaplan, H.S.: Hodgkin's disease: Unfolding concepts concerning its nature, management and prognosis. *Cancer* 45:2439–2474, 1980.

Mitchel, R.I., Peters, M.V.: Lymph node biopsy during laparotomy for the staging of Hodgkin's disease. *Ann. Surg.* 178:698–702, 1973.

Panettiere, F., Coltman, C.A.: Splenectomy effects on chemotherapy in Hodgkin's disease. *Arch. Intern. Med.* 131:362–366, 1973.

Salzman, J.R., Kaplan, H.S.: Effect of prior splenectomy on hematologic tolerance during total lymphoid radiotherapy of patients with Hodgkin's disease. *Cancer* 27:471–478, 1971.

Sandusky, W.R., Jones, R.C.W., Horsley, J.S., et al: Staging laparotomy in Hodgkin's disease. *Ann. Surg.* 187:485–489, 1978.

Schimpff, S.C., O'Connell, N.J., Greene, W.H., et al.: Infections in ninety-two splenectomized patients with Hodgkin's disease: A clinical review. *Am. J. Med.* 9:695–701, 1975.

Sutcliffe, S.B.J., Bansfeld, T.A., Wrigley, T.F.M., et al.: Post treatment laparotomy in the management of Hodgkin's disease. *Lancet* 2:57–60, 1978.

Sutcliffe, S.B.J., Wrigley, P.F.M., Smyth, J.F., et al.: Intensive investigation in management of Hodgkin's disease. *Br. Med. J.* 2:1343–1347, 1976.

Sweet, D.L., Kinnealey, A., Ultmann, J.E.: Hodgkin's disease: Problems of staging. *Cancer* 42:957–970, 1978.

Veronesi, U., Nusumeci, R., Pizzetti, F., et al.: The value of staging laparotomy in non-Hodgkin's lymphomas. *Cancer* 33:446–459, 1974.

Whittaker, J.A., Slater, A., Al-Ismail, S.A.B., et al.: An assessment of laparotomy in the management of patients with Hodgkin's disease. *Q. J. Med.* New Series XLVII, 187:291–301, 1978.

5

Lymphomas of the Gastrointestinal Tract

John G. Allison, M.D.

Introduction

Lymphomatous involvement of the stomach, small bowel, and colon may be primary, arising from the lymphoid tissue in the gut, or secondary, associated with disseminated systemic lymphoma of the non-Hodgkin's type. Secondary spread of non-Hodgkin's lymphoma (NHL) to the gastrointestinal tract is usually hematogenous, although direct spread by contiguity from other organs may occur and is the more common occurrence in Hodgkin's disease. Lymphomas arising primarily in the stomach, small bowel, and colon have a metastatic progression similar to that seen with the more frequent epithelial carcinomas and may spread by continuity within the organ, by contiguity to adjacent organs, via the lymphatics to local and then regional lymph nodes, and finally via the blood stream. Transcelomic or intraluminal spread has not been reported.

It is of critical importance to make the distinction between primary and secondary involvement of the gut by lymphoma because of the substantial difference in natural history, treatment, and prognosis. The secondary, or metastatic, lymphoma is usually a late manifestation of widely disseminated disease, is frequently multifocal, and invariably places the patient in Stage IV. Surgical intervention is reserved for the complications of obstruction, perforation, and hemorrhage, in contrast with the primary lymphomas in which resection of the disease can be of major therapeutic benefit. Treatment of secondary involvement of the gut must perforce be systemic, with judicious use of radiotherapy for bulky disease. Radiotherapy, however, plays a major role as an adjunct to resection of the primary lymphomas, with chemotherapy usually having been reserved for salvage in the event of wide dissemination or recurrence. There are early and tantalizing data, however, to suggest that chemotherapy alone may equal, or exceed, the long-term survival in Stages I and II (Ann Arbor) NHL of the aggressive histological subtype and this experience may well be extrapolated to the primary gastrointestinal lymphomas in the future. This refers especially to those instances where the disease has spread to lymph nodes or to adjacent organs. Many would still agree that surgical extirpation is required in Stage I lymphoma but that chemotherapy will replace radiation therapy (with its attendant risks when the abdomen is irradiated) as the optimal adjuvant.

Primary lymphomas of the gastrointestinal tract arise in the lymphoid tissue scattered throughout the submucosa of the bowel. The possible relationship between a difference in the recirculation and migration properties of lymphoid cells having their origin in the gut and those arising in other lymphoreticular sites, and the more favorable outlook associated with primary gut lymphomas, has been summarized by Blackledge et al. Other prognostic factors are the site of origin (gastric having the best survival and colorectal the worst), the growth pattern of the individual lymphoma (nodular being more favorable than diffuse), and the extent of regional nodal spread or invasion of contiguous organs. Sixteen reports, encompassing 1,110 patients, of primary gastrointestinal tract lymphomas were reviewed; the results are summarized in Table 1.

Within this review, the lymphocytic lymphomas comprise a little over one-half (52%) and include a wide spectrum of all subtypes in this group. Forty-two percent were of the histiocytic variety, although this rather large proportion is influenced somewhat by the predominance of primary gastric tumors, of which 57% are histiocytic lymphomas. The remaining 6% include those of mixed histology, those in which definite histological variety could not be specified, and Hodgkin's disease. The more recent literature would suggest, however, that the histiocytic lymphomas are more common than previously believed, and may actually be more common than the lymphocytic variety. Closer histopathological scrutiny with newer techniques is likely to account for this changing distribution. Whereas it was previously thought that approximately 5% of primary gastrointestinal tract lymphomas were Hodgkin's disease, this concept has been challenged by Henry and Farrer-Brown who believe that a diagnosis of primary Hodgkin's disease of the gut is a spurious one. It is possible that in the past, multinucleated giant cells have been confused with Reed-Sternberg cells, resulting in a wrong histopathological label.

Table 1
Data from 16 Reports* (1,110 patients) on Site and Histological Type of Primary Gastrointestinal Lymphoma

	Number of Patients	Determinate Patients	Percent
Gastric	578	1110	52
Small bowel**	430	1110	39
Colorectal	102	1110	9
Lymphocytic	391	759	52
Histiocytic	318	759	42
Other***	50	759	5

*Not all reports adequately expressed histology, hence the discrepancy in "determinate" patients.
**Includes duodenum, ileocecum, and appendix.
***Includes mixed, undifferentiated, and Hodgkin's disease.

Plasma cell elements in these alimentary tract lymphomas are being recognized more frequently, and the incidence of plasmacytoma of the gastrointestinal tract is being reported in 4–39% of nonepithelial and nonmesenchymal neoplasms. These plasma cell tumors are infrequently associated with a monoclonal peak on plasma electrophoresis, and care must be exercised to distinguish the primary isolated extramedullary plasmacytoma from an extramedullary lesion associated with multiple myeloma, as the management and prognosis of the two are different. It is currently not fully understood whether this plasma cell element is an antecedent phenomenon or whether it represents differentiation into an immunoblastic type of lymphoma. Lymphomas of the stomach, small bowel, and colon constitute approximately 1% of all the malignant neoplasms involving the GI tract, the small bowel having the highest ratio (to carcinoma) and the colon and rectum the lowest.

Seventy-five to 80% of lymphomas involving the gastrointestinal tract will be primary, with 75% of these being solitary. Multifocal and disseminated primary disease will be seen in 20% and 5%, respectively. When primary and secondary lesions are considered together, there is an equal distribution of approximately 40% each between stomach and small bowel. Only 15–20% arise in, or secondarily involve, the colon or rectum.

Because of the different site of origin, mode of spread, and natural behavior, the application of the Ann Arbor staging may not be appropriate. Many have suggested using a staging method similar to that described by Dukes for rectal carcinoma, in which Stage I implies disease confined to the bowel wall without penetration of the serosa; Stage II, penetration of the serosa without nodal or metastatic disease; Stage III, regional nodal disease; and Stage IV, distant nodal or metastatic disease. Others have recommended the use of a TNM system, with the stages based on scoring for the extent of tumor involvement and for nodal and metastatic disease. The TNM categories for adenocarcinoma of the stomach are outlined in Table 2, and the adaptation for application to gastric lymphoma, as suggested by Lim et al., in Table 3. Because of the different behavior and the greater propensity for nodal spread, I have exercised a little editorial license and modified both by including an N3 status to include distal nodal metastases, as these may not carry the dire prognostic significance that they do with an epithelial carcinoma.

Table 2
Definitions of TNM Categories (Gastric Carcinoma—Adapted for Lymphoma)

T—Primary tumor
- T_1—Confined to the mucosa
- T_2—Involves the mucosa, the submucosa including the muscularis propria, and extends to, or into, the serosa but does not penetrate the serosa
- T_3—Penetrates through the serosa with or without invasion of contiguous structures
- T_4*—Diffusely involves the entire thickness of the stomach wall without obvious boundaries (including linitis plastica)
- T_x—Degree of penetration of stomach wall not determined

N—Regional lymph nodes
- N_0—No metastasis to nodes
- N_1—Metastasis to the perigastric lymph nodes in the immediate vicinity of the primary tumor
- N_2—Metastasis to the perigastric lymph nodes at a distance from the primary tumor or on both curvatures of the stomach, or to the splenic hilar, suprapancreatic, or celiac axis groups of nodes
- N_3**—Metastasis to distant lymph nodes, e.g., mediastinal

M—Distant metastasis
- M_0—No distant metastasis
- M_1—Clinical, roentgenographic, or operative evidence of distant metastasis (for carcinoma, includes nodes beyond the regional lymph nodes) but excluding direct extension in contiguity by the primary tumor

*It is unlikely that this category exists for primary lymphoma of the gut, with the possible (but not widely accepted) exception of the "Mediterranean" small bowel lymphoma.

**Author's suggested modification for lymphoma; this replaces the inclusion of distant nodal metastasis in the category M_1 for epithelial cancer.

Table 3
TNM Staging (Gastric Carcinoma—Adapted for Lymphoma)

Stage I	A	T_1	N_0	M_0
	B	T_2	N_0	M_0
	C	T_3	N_0	M_0
Stage II*	A	T_{1-3}	N_1	M_0
Stage III*	A	T_{1-4}	N_2	M_0
	B	T_{1-4}	N_3	M_0
Stage IV		Any T or N with M_1		

*Author's modifications: Stage II is not subdivided into A and B and no N_3 exists in Stage III for epithelial cancers.

Lack of consistency in the literature in assessing stage renders meaningful analysis of survival according to stage impossible. The impact of local spread and nodal and distant metastases will be discussed in the sections dealing with the individual anatomical sites of origin. Gastrointestinal lymphomas may be found in any age group, but the peak incidence is in the sixth and seventh decades, with a slight male preponderance. There is a smaller peak in children under the age of 12 years with a very distinct male preponderance (9:1 in one series) and involving almost exclusively the small bowel; there is a considerable predominance of the diffuse undifferentiated subtype in these children.

Primary Gastric Lymphoma

Of all the primary gastrointestinal lymphomas, those arising in the stomach have the best prognosis. Survival rates are substantially better than those for adenocarcinoma of the stomach and therefore any patient with a primary gastric tumor, in whom a preoperative histological diagnosis of lymphoma cannot be excluded, deserves an exploratory laparotomy. With the sophistication of endoscopic biopsies, brush biopsies, and cytology on gastric washings, confusion is less likely to occur than has been reported in the past. As almost 5% of malignant neoplasms arising in the stomach are lymphomatous, failure to acquire a tissue diagnosis places an obligation on the surgeon to perform a diagnostic laparotomy if a potentially retrievable situation is to be recognized.

The clinical manifestation of a gastric lymphoma may mimic very closely those of benign gastric ulceration and carcinoma. Abdominal pain is the most common feature and may be the presenting symptom in 70–90% of patients. About one-half of patients will experience anorexia and nausea, these two symptoms invariably being associated with a substantial loss of weight. Ten to 20% have a clinically detectable abdominal mass at the time of presentation. Evidence of gastric outlet obstruction, such as early satiety and vomiting, are functions of the size and location of the tumor, being obviously more common in the bulkier lesions arising more distally in the stomach. Although bleeding and perforation do occur, the incidence is less than that with either benign gastric ulcer or carcinoma. Fewer than 10% can be expected to have a concomitant anemia, resulting from chronic blood loss, at the time of diagnosis. Jaundice is rare but, when present, is usually obstructive and due to extrinsic compression of the common bile duct by large nodal metastases in the porta hepatis.

The progression of diagnostic evaluation will include certain routine investigations (chest and abdominal roentgenograms, a full blood count, and serological tests of liver function) followed by upper gastrointestinal contrast roentgenograms and endoscopy. It may be impossible to distinguish a gastric lymphoma from a gastric carcinoma on the upper GI series, although subtle discriminating features have been described. These include multiple filling defects, large tumors inappropriate to the general condition of the patient, a large tumor with relatively normal pliability of the rest of the stomach, hypertrophic, thickened, and often polypoid-appearing rugae associated with the mass, and deep excavating ulcers. It is nevertheless usually impossible to make the distinction. Endoscopy, using a fiberoptic instrument, with multiple biopsies will frequently resolve the issue. Cytological evaluation is less sensitive. Without special staining techniques or immunocytochemistry, isolated lymphoma cells may be indistinguishable from those of a poorly differentiated or undifferentiated malignancy of epithelial origin, and making a definite diagnosis may be extremely difficult. Subtyping on cytology alone is certainly impossible.

If a primary lymphoma is suspected, the routine use of bone marrow biopsies is probably not indicated and should probably be reserved for evaluation of dissemination when widely extensive disease is discovered at laparotomy. Radionuclide scanning does not appear to be used as frequently, or have any value, with the primary lymphomas. A CAT scan may provide information on nodal and visceral metastatic disease in both the abdomen and the thorax that may influence decisions regarding the use and selection of adjunctive therapy but it is unlikely to influence the decision for exploratory laparotomy. All patients with primary gastric lymphoma merit exploration as the resectability rate is high and even palliative resections may provide up to 25% 5-year survival rates. Treatment of primary gastric lymphoma by radiation therapy alone is attended by a very low long-term survival. Gastric resection, with or without adjunctive radiotherapy, provides the best results and remains the treatment of choice.

The extent of resection in both carcinoma and lymphoma of the stomach is controversial. There is evidence, however, to suggest that wide lymphadenectomy as part of an extended radical total gastrectomy, to include the spleen and its hilar nodes, the tail of the pancreas, and the suprapancreatic nodes, does improve survival in early (Stages I and II) adenocarcinoma of the stomach. Whether this principle, in truth, applies to lymphoma is uncertain, but Connors and Wise and ReMine advocate total gastrectomy as part of a radical and aggressive resection to improve survival. Furthermore, detection of nodal metastases in what might otherwise be considered an early stage lymphoma may be a decisive factor leading to postoperative irradiation. In this role it may perhaps be regarded as a staging procedure. Additional arguments favoring total gastrectomy over segmental resections are a 60% incidence of multifocality and a 10% incidence of diffuse infiltration of the gastric wall. With improved preoperative and postoperative care and the advent of circular stapling devices, a total gastrectomy with esophagojejunal anastomosis is no longer fraught with the horrendous mortality and morbidity experienced 30 or more years ago. There are many, nevertheless, who believe that a subtotal gastric resection is adequate.

Although the extent of resection may be controversial, there exists a consensus that long-term survival is definitely improved by the use of adjunctive radiation therapy, especially in TNM Stages II and IIIA. The comments made earlier in this chapter concerning the potential for chemotherapy replacing radiation therapy certainly apply (as they do to subsequent discussions on the treatment of small bowel and colorectal lymphoma) but there is scant evidence that the turning point has arrived.

In their comprehensive literature review of 2,400 patients with gastric lymphoma, Brooks and Enterline found the statistically significant favorable prognostic variables to be Stage I disease, smaller tumor size (less than 7 cm), and only superficial gastric wall invasion. The overall tendency for lymphomas of the lymphocytic type and those with a nodular growth pattern to have a better prognosis was noted, although this did not achieve statistical significance. The 5-year survival rate (for all stages) was 40%, with little further change at 10 years, suggesting that few die of their disease after 5 years. Five-year survival rates of up to 88% have been reported in the absence of serosal penetration or nodal metastases which, in that particular series, reduced survival to 24% and 32%, respectively.

The role of single or multiagent chemotherapy in the treatment of primary gastric lymphoma has not been elucidated. It would seem logical, however, that chemotherapy would have an important place in the management of primary lymphomas when they are multifocal, not amenable to resection, and when radiotherapy is impracticable.

In summary, the outlook for patients with primary gastric lymphoma is less bleak than that for those with other primary epithelial or mesenchymal malignant neoplasms. Successful treatment, and hence long-term survival, is nevertheless predicated by the earlier diagnosis of early disease. Wide gastric resection with a generous lymphadenectomy should be performed for both therapeutic and prognostic reasons. With the exception of Stage I disease (where its advantage seems to be marginal) adjunctive radiation therapy of at least 2,500 rads should be administered.

No discussion of lymphoma of the stomach would be complete without addressing the interesting entity of pseudolymphoma. This is an uncommon benign condition, although it has been suggested by some that it may represent a premalignant phase of primary gastric lymphoma. It has been reported as occurring in other organs including lung, lacrimal gland, parotid, and skin.

The primary histological distinguishing features between pseudolymphoma and malignant lymphoma are the formation of follicles with true germinal centers and the absence of lymph node involvement. The pseudolymphomas are always of the lymphocytic cell type. Additional features are those of a nodular architecture with an inflammatory infiltrate, predominantly polymorphonuclear. Mitotic figures are infrequent and, when present, are confined to reaction centers. The pseudolymphomas tend to be well localized with no submucosal infiltration and are invariably ulcerated.

They may prove to be diagnostic and therapeutic dilemmas because of the confusion with gastric adenocarcinoma or primary lymphoma. The clinical presentation closely mimics that of benign gastric ulcer or ulcerating gastric carcinoma, although the duration of symptoms may be somewhat longer. The main symptom complex includes abdominal pain and nausea, with vomiting being fairly frequent. Although perforation is rare, the complication of upper gastrointestinal hemorrhage, presenting as hematemesis and melena, or with anemia resulting from chronic blood loss, does occur. The radiological and endoscopic appearances are indistinguishable from those of a carcinoma or benign ulcer; the association of a large ulcerated mass with thickened and distorted mucosal rugae is suggestive. Benign ulcers are usually associated with an atrophic gastritis, while effacement of the rugal folds due to submucosal infiltration is more characteristic of malignant disease, both adenocarcinoma and malignant lymphoma. Endoscopic biopsy may be unreliable in making a definitive diagnosis, which is usually confirmed by histopathological examination of the resected stomach. The treatment of choice is subtotal gastric resection. No adjunctive treatment is necessary and, as the condition is benign, the prognosis is excellent. The premalignant potential of gastric pseudolymphoma remains an unproven theory and its etiological origin remains obscure. Although commonly associated with ulceration, the concept that a gastric pseudolymphoma is a response to benign gastric ulceration is also not widely accepted. Most, but not all, are associated with ulceration and it is rare for the pseudolymphomatous changes to extend beyond the ulceration-scarring process. Furthermore, they have been found in association with achlorhydria and, as mentioned, reported in organs in which ulceration does not occur.

Suffice it to say that the distinction between pseudolymphoma and lymphoma of the stomach is important, as the patient may be spared a radical gastric resection and needs undergo neither irradiation nor chemotherapy.

Lymphoma of the Small Bowel

Primary lymphomatous involvement of the small bowel presents an interesting spectrum of disease. There are several variants, each of which appears to have its own particular epidemiology, behavior, associated disorders, and prognosis. These variants are the so-called "Mediterranean" lymphoma, the "Western" lymphoma, and American (or abdominal) Burkitt's lymphoma. Because of the site of origin these small bowel lymphomas are of B-cell derivation; any lymphoma, apparently of T-cell origin, should be regarded with great suspicion and a primary vigorously sought for elsewhere.

Mediterranean Lymphoma

This rather fascinating subgroup of primary small bowel lymphoma was termed "Mediterranean" lymphoma because of the high prevalence in Middle Eastern countries, including Israel, affecting Arabs and Jews. Within the Jewish population, it is almost exclusively the non-European (Sephardic) Jews that develop the disease, while Jews of European origin (Ashkenazi) are spared. The incidence in Arabs living within Israel is higher than that in Arabs living elsewhere. The term "Mediterranean," however, may shortly become obsolete as several cases have subsequently been reported in Blacks and those of mixed ethnic origin in South Africa, and sporadic cases have surfaced in North America.

This "Mediterranean" lymphoma is a disease of young adults and children, most of the cases being male. The proximal small bowel (duodenum and jejunum) is the site in which this variant occurs. The histopathological features of the Mediterranean lymphoma contrast very strikingly with those of the Western type. A dominant histological feature of the former is a dense plasma cell infiltration which usually extends well beyond the limits of frank lymphoma. Widespread and marked villous atrophy is a characteristic feature, often associated with crypt hyperplasia, and these patients invariably present with diarrhea and malabsorption. Other changes that have been noted in the epithelium are those of loss of basal orientation of the nuclei, pseudostratification, and an increased number of intraepithelial lymphocytes. In areas where the bowel is infiltrated with a frank lymphoma, the histology may be that of a bizarre pleomorphic spectrum of cells ranging from atypical lymphocytes to large cells of the histiocytic variety which may even resemble Reed-Sternberg cells.

A fascinating feature of the Mediterranean lymphoma is the association with α-heavy chain disease, in which an unusual type of abnormal immunoglobulin is found in various body fluids. This abnormal protein is closely related to the Fc fragment of immunoglobulin A (IgA) and is deficient in the light (λ) chains. There have been isolated cases reported in which free α-chains have been identified in the serum and urine. Abnormalities of the other immunoglobulin fractions have been documented, with increases in IgM and decreases in IgG. The immunoblastic origin of these lymphomas is supported by the finding of all major immunoglobulin classes within the malignant cells of single tumors, irrespective of the histological appearances. The association of the "plasmacytoid" infiltration with these lymphomas is obscure. There have been patients who, on peroral jejunal biopsies, have demonstrated this infiltration in association with α-heavy chain disease but who have not manifested with a frank lymphoma. This has led to the suggestion that the diffuse plasma cell infiltrate may be the primary pathology, having a strong malignant potential. It is unlikely that it represents a cellular response, as has been suggested by some, to a primary lymphoma. An attempt to explain away the presence of the plasma cells as part of a differentiation or dedifferentiation process has not gained much support, nor has the suggestion that all these tumors be labeled "plasmacytomas" gained much popularity. Because of the epidemiology, particularly the geographical influence, there is a strong belief that environmental factors play an important part in the etiology of the Mediterranean lymphoma, although a genetic trait has also been invoked.

Radiation therapy or multiagent chemotherapy, or a combination of the two, is the treatment of choice for the Mediterranean lymphoma, with surgery generally being reserved for complications of obstruction, perforation, or hemorrhage. Because of the diffuse intramural extent of the lymphomatous deposits and plasma cell infiltrate, radical and devastating surgery would be required. The role of primary chemotherapy in this disease is promising and has been used in several institutions for the treatment of late or recurrent disease. The overall 2-year survival rate appears to be approximately 20%, the primary determinant of survival being the stage of the disease at the time of diagnosis. The Mediterranean lymphoma, unfortunately, seems to spread early through the serosa and to local and regional lymph nodes, thus prejudicing the outcome. There are but a few patients in Stage II, and almost none in Stage III or IV, who survive beyond 2 years.

Western Lymphoma

The "Western" type of small bowel lymphoma has a very different pathology, behavior, clinical presentation, and prognosis. These occur later in life, with the peak influence in the fifth decade, and have a slight male preponderance.

The majority (almost two-thirds) of these are lymphocytic lymphomas and occur in the distal small bowel. These more commonly present as a manifestation of tumor bulk with an abdominal mass or distal small bowel obstruction. Perforation and hemorrhage are infrequent.

Prognosis and survival are superior to those associated with Mediterranean lymphoma and surgical resection plays a much more important role in the therapy. Wherever possible a wide resection encompassing all local lymph node groups should be effected. Frozen section examination of margins should be obtained. Failure to gain a free histological margin prejudices survival. Adjunctive radiation therapy of at least 2,000 rads has become accepted as an important factor in significantly improving survival. There has been little place for chemotherapy other than for widely disseminated disease (e.g., to bone marrow or liver) or as a palliative measure for recurrence, although the future may see a greater emphasis put on this modality. Overall 5-year survival rates may attain 40% but, once again, stage at time of diagnosis is a critical factor. No patients having palliative resections, with or without irradiation or chemotherapy, have survived this period.

American Burkitt's lymphoma is a disease primarily of children and young adults, with a peak incidence in the late teens. About one-half of the patients will already have extraabdominal disease at the time of diagnosis and consequently a much poorer prognosis. An abdominal mass or intestinal obstruction (often due to intussusception) is the usual mode of presentation—a correct preoperative diagnosis is seldom made.

When the disease appears to be localized, an attempted curative resection, followed by adjunctive chemotherapy and abdominal irradiation, provides a much better long-term prognosis (nearly 60% 5-year survival) than simple biopsy or incomplete resection. This difference may, in part, reflect the mortality from complications (perforation and hemorrhage) which result from the rapid tumor dissolution, a characteristic response of Burkitt's lymphoma to chemotherapy. An aggressive surgical approach is thus recommended whenever practical.

Primary distal small bowel lymphoma has been reported as occurring in patients with inflammatory bowel disease (Crohn's disease), but other than a possible common association with abnormalities of the immune system, no cause or effect relationship has been identified. The two may easily be confused on roentgenographic contrast studies (enteroclysis).

Another interesting association is that with adult celiac disease. Recurrence of symptoms (diarrhea and malabsorption) in those who have responded to and remained well on a gluten-free diet should rouse suspicions that the change in status is due to the appearance of a lymphoma. Adult celiac disease is characterized by a lymphopenia, particularly of the T-cell population, which may bear a relationship to the development of lymphoma. A further decrease in the lymphocyte count may herald the advent of a small bowel lymphoma in these patients, and a mass lesion in the presence of the typical mucosal changes on enteroclysis would be highly suggestive.

Lymphoma of the Colon and Rectum

These are the least common areas in which primary gastrointestinal tract lymphomas are found (approximately 0.3% of colorectal tumors). The majority are of the lymphocytic variety and multifocality is a common feature. There have been several reports of primary colonic lymphoma (histiocytic) arising in patients who have long-standing chronic ulcerative colitis, but other than a possible association similar to that seen with Crohn's disease and small bowel lymphoma, no specific relationship has been documented. Colonic lymphoma may closely mimic ulcerative colitis and there are patients who have mistakenly been treated for the latter condition for several years. The roentgenographic and endoscopic appearances of the two may be indistinguishable and the histological appearances of biopsy specimens may be inconclusive. The issue of whether or not ulcerative colitis truly represents a "prelymphoma" state has not been resolved.

Because of the larger diameter and greater distensibility of the colon, unless the colonic lymphomas present with bleeding, the diagnosis is usually made late. Perforation or invasion of adjacent structures may be the presenting features and both carry grave prognostic implications. Bleeding, diarrhea, and tenesmus are common with rectal lymphomas.

When present as a mass lesion, a colonic lymphoma may have an identical appearance to that of an adenocarcinoma, and may also resemble an "apple-core" lesion. The most characteristic feature on barium enema is a diffuse nodularity of the mucosa, which, in the presence of symptoms, should always be regarded with suspicion.

Resection and adjunctive radiation therapy is the treatment of choice for both colonic and rectal lesions. Overall 5-year survival rate is low, approximately 15–20%, and reflects the later stage at which these tumors present, although a 55% 5-year survival has been reported for rectal lymphoma treated with radical surgery and post-operative radiation therapy.

Selected Reading

Al-Saleem, T., Al-Bahrani, Z.: Lymphoma of the small intestine in Iraq (Middle East lymphoma). *Cancer* 31:291–294, 1973.

Anderson, J.R., Lee, D., Naysmith, A., et al.: Gastric pseudolymphoma. *Br. J. Surg.* 67:672–674, 1980.

Bedikian, A.Y., Khankhanian, N., Heilbrun, L.K., et al.: Primary lymphomas and sarcomas of the stomach. *Southern Med. J.* 73:21–24, 1980.

Blackledge, G., Bush, H., Dodge, O.G., et al.: A study of gastrointestinal lymphoma. *Clin. Oncol.* 5:209–219, 1979.

Bonomo, L., Dammacco, F., Marano, R., et al.: Abdominal lymphoma and alpha-chain disease. Report of 3 cases. *Am. J. Med.* 52:73–86, 1972.

Borochovitz, D., Dutz, W., Kohout, E., et al.: Gastrointestinal mucosa and primary gastrointestinal lymphoma. *Israel J. Med. Sci.* 15:397–404, 1979.

Brandt, L., Hagander, B., Norden, A., et al.: Lymphoma of the small intestine in adult celiac disease. *Med. Scand.* 204:467–470, 1978.

Brooks, J.J., Enterline, H.T.: Gastric pseudolymphoma: Its three subtypes and relation to lymphoma. *Cancer* 51:476–486, 1983.

Brooks, J.J., Enterline, H.T.: Primary gastric lymphomas: A clinicopathologic study of 58 cases with long-term followup and literature review. *Cancer* 51:701–711, 1983.

Bush, R.S., Ash, C.L.: Primary lymphoma of the gastrointestinal tract. *Radiology* 92:1349–1354, 1959.

Cabanillas, F., Bodey, G.P., Freireich, E.J.: Management with chemotherapy only of Stage I and II malignant lymphoma of aggressive histologic types. *Cancer* 46:2356–2359, 1980.

Chiles, J.T., Platz, C.E.: The radiographic manifestations of pseudolymphoma of the stomach. *Radiology* 116:551–556, 1975.

Cohen, H.J., Gonzalvo, A., Krook, J., et al.: New presentation of alpha-heavy-chain disease: North American polypoid gastrointestinal lymphoma. Clinical and cellular studies. *Cancer* 41:1161–1169, 1978.

Connors, J., Wise, L.: Management of gastric lymphomas. *Am. J. Surg.* 127:102–108, 1974.

Contreary, K., Nance, F.C., Becker, W.F.: Primary lymphoma of the gastrointestinal tract. *Ann. Surg.* 191:593–598, 1980.

Craig, O., Gregson, R.: Primary lymphoma of the gastrointestinal tract. *Clin. Radiol.* 32:63–71, 1981.

Cupps, R.E., Hodgson, J.R., Dockerty, M.B., et al.: Primary lymphoma in the small intestine: Problems of roentgenologic diagnosis. *Radiology* 92:1355–1362, 1969.

Fleming, I.D., Mitchell, S., Dilawari, R.A.: The role of surgery in the management of gastric lymphoma. *Cancer* 49:1135–1141, 1982.

Freeman, H.G., Weinstein, W.M., Shnitka, P.K., et al.: Primary abdominal lymphoma. Presenting manifestations of celiac sprue or complicating dermatitis herpetiformis. *Am. J. Med.* 63:585–594, 1977.

Friedman, H.B., Silver, G.M., Brown, C.H.: Lymphoma of the colon simulating ulcerative colitis. Report of 4 cases. *Am. J. Digest. Dis.* 13:910–917, 1968.

Fu, Y.-S., Perzin, K.H.: Lymphosarcoma of the small intestine: A clinicopathologic study. *Cancer* 29:645–659, 1972.

Green, J.A., Dawson, A.A., Lessells, A.M., et al.: Prognostic factors in gastrointestinal lymphoma. *Clin. Oncol.* 7:115–121, 1981.

Gupta, S., Pant, G.C., Gupta, S.: A clinicopathological study of primary gastrointestinal lymphoma. *J. Surg. Oncol.* 16:49–58, 1981.

Haghighi, P., Kharazmi, A., Gerami, C., et al.: Primary upper small intestinal lymphoma and alpha-chain disease. Report of 10 cases emphasizing pathological aspects. *Am. J. Surg. Pathol.* 2:147–157, 1978.

Hande, K.R., Fisher, R.I., DeVita, V.T., et al.: Diffuse histiocytic lymphoma involving the gastrointestinal tract. *Cancer* 41:1984–1989, 1978.

Hermann, R., Panahon, A.M., Barcos, N.P., et al.: Gastrointestinal involvement in non-Hodgkin's lymphoma. *Cancer* 46:215–222, 1980.

Highman, L.M., Fantelli, F.J., Hermann, R.E.: Pseudolymphoma of the stomach. *Arch. Surg.* 116:227–229, 1981.

Ho, F., Gibson, J.B.: Gastrointestinal lymphomas in Hong Kong Chinese. *Israel J. Med. Sci.* 15:382–385, 1979.

Hoerr, S.O., McCormack, L.J., Hertzer, N.R.: Prognosis in gastric lymphoma. *Arch. Surg.* 107:155–158, 1973.

Ike, V.W., Rosenbusch, G.: Gastrointestinal malignant lymphoma: Roentgenographic features and pathologic and morphologic correlations. *Diagnostic Imaging* 50:66–80, 1981.

Isaacson, P., Wright, D.H.: Intestinal lymphoma associated with malabsorption. *Lancet* 1:67–70, 1978.

Isaacson, P., Wright, D.H., Judd, M.A., et al.: Primary gastrointestinal lymphomas: A classification of 66 cases. *Cancer* 43:1805–1819, 1979.

Kahn, L.B., Novis, B.H.: Nodular lymphoid hyperplasia of the small bowel associated with primary small bowel reticulum cell lymphoma. *Cancer* 33:837–844, 1974.

Kahn, L.D., Selzer, G., Kaschula, R.O.C.: Primary gastrointestinal lymphoma: A clinicopathologic study of 57 cases. *Digest. Dis.* 17:219–232, 1972.

Kemeny, M.M., Magrath, I.T., Brennan, N.F.: The role of surgery in the management of American Burkitt's lymphoma and its treatment. *Ann. Surg.* 196:82–86, 1982.

Khojasteh, A., Haghshenass, M., Haghighi, P.: Immunoproliferative small intestinal disease. *N. Engl. J. Med.* 308:1401–1405, 1983.

Kopec, M., Swierczylska, Z., Pazdur, J., et al.: Diffuse lymphoma of the intestines with a monoclonal gammopathy of IgG_3 kappa type. *Am. J. Med.* 56:381–385, 1974.

Lee, H.Y., Cogbill, C.L.: Primary lymphosarcoma of the stomach. *Am. Surg.* 37:256–262, 1971.

Lewin, K.J., Kahn, L.B., Novis, B.H.: Primary intestinal lymphomas of "Western" and "Mediterranean" type. Alpha-chain disease and massive plasma cell infiltration. A comparative study of 37 cases. *Cancer* 38:2511–2528, 1976.

Lewin, K.J., Ranchod, M., Dorfman, R.F.: Lymphomas of the gastrointestinal tract: A study of 117 cases presenting with gastrointestinal disease. *Cancer* 42:693–707, 1978.

Lim, F.E., Hartman, A.S., Tan, E.G.C., et al.: Factors in the prognosis of gastric lymphoma. *Cancer* 39:1715–1720, 1977.

Loehr, W.J., Mujahed, Z., Zahn, F.D., et al.: Primary lymphoma of the gastrointestinal tract: A review of 100 cases. *Ann. Surg.* 170:232–238, 1969.

Mattingly, S.S., Sibull, M.L., Ram, M.D., et al.: Pseudolymphoma of the stomach. A diagnostic and therapeutic dilemma. *Arch. Surg.* 116:25–29, 1981.

Naqvi, M.S., Burrows, L., Kark, A.E.: Lymphoma of the gastrointestinal tract: Prognostic guides based on 162 cases. *Ann. Surg.* 170:221–231, 1969.

Nasr, K., Haghighi, P., Bakshandeh, K., et al.: Primary lymphoma of the upper small intestine. *Gut* 11:673–678, 1970.

Nasr, K., Haghighi, P., Bakshandeh, K., et al.: Primary upper small intestinal lymphoma: A report of 40 cases from Iran. *Digest. Dis.* 21:313–323, 1976.

Nelson, D.F., Cassady, J.R., Traggis, B., et al.: The role of radiation therapy in localized resectable intestinal non-Hodgkin's lymphoma in children. *Cancer* 39:89–97, 1977.

Novak, S., Caraveo, J., Trowbridge, A.A., et al.: Primary lymphomas of the gastrointestinal tract. *Southern Med. J.* 72:1154–1158, 1979.

Novis B.H.: Primary intestinal lymphoma in South Africa. *Israel J. Med. Sci.* 15:386–389, 1979.

Novis, B.H., Bank, S., Marks, I.N., et al.: Abdominal lymphoma presenting with malabsorption. *Q. J. Med.* 40:521–540, 1971.

O'Connell, D.J., Thompson, A.J.: Lymphoma of the colon: The spectrum of radiologic changes. *Gastroint. Radiol.* 2:377–385, 1978.

Otto, H.F., Bettmann, I., von Weltzien, J., et al.: Primary intestinal lymphomas. *Virchows Arch.* (*Pathol. Anat.*) 391:9–31, 1981.

Perry, P.M., Cross, R.M., Morson, B.C.: Primary malignant lymphoma of the rectum (22 cases). *Proc. Roy. Soc. Med.* 65:8, 1972.

Privett, J.T.J., Davies, E.R., Roylance, J.: The radiological features of gastric lymphoma. *Clin. Radiol.* 28:457–463, 1977.

Radaszkiewicz, T., Dragosics, B.: Primary lymphomas of the gastrointestinal tract: A clinicopathologic study of 60 cases. *Pathol. Res. Pract.* 169:363–365, 1980.

Ramot, B., Many, A.: Primary intestinal lymphoma: Clinical manifestations and possible effect of environmental factors. *Recent Results Cancer Res.* 39:193–199, 1972.

Rappaport, H., Ramot, B., Hulu, N., et al.: The pathology of so-called Mediterranean abdominal lymphoma with malabsorption. *Cancer* 29:1502–1511, 1972.

Salnelah, H.: Lymphosarcoma of the stomach: A clinical study of 39 cases. *Acta Chir. Scand.* 134:567–576, 1968.

Selzer, G., Sacks, M., Sherman, G., et al.: Primary malignant lymphoma of the small intestine in Israel: Changing incidence with time. *Israel J. Med. Sci.* 15:390–396, 1979.

Selzer, G., Sherman, G., Callihan, T.R., et al.: Primary small intestinal lymphomas and alpha-heavy-chain disease: A study of 43 cases from a pathology department in Israel. *Israel J. Med. Sci.* 15:111–123, 1979.

Shahid, M.J., Alami, S.Y., Nassar, V.H., et al.: Primary intestinal lymphoma with paraproteinemia. *Cancer* 35:848–858, 1975.

Shiu, M.H., Kras, M., Nisce, L., et al.: Management of primary gastric lymphoma. *Ann. Surg.* 195:196–202, 1981.

Stroehlein, J.R., Weiland, L.H., Hoffman, H.M., et al.: Untreated gastric pseudolymphoma. *Digest. Dis.* 22:465–470, 1977.

Wagonfeld, J.B., Platz, C.E., Fishman, F.L., et al.: Multicentric colonic lymphoma complicating ulcerative colitis. *Digest Dis.* 22:502–508, 1977.

Weingrad, D.N., Decosse, J.J., Sherlock, P., et al.: Primary gastrointestinal lymphoma: A 30-year review. *Cancer* 49:1258–1265, 1982.

Zornoza, J., Dodd, G.D.: Lymphoma of the gastrointestinal tract. *Semin. Roentgenol.* 15:272–287, 1980.

6

Chemotherapy of the Lymphomas

James O. Armitage, M.D.

Introduction

The lymphomas can be thought of in three broad groups for therapeutic considerations (see Table 1). Patients with Hodgkin's disease are generally younger, often have localized disease that can be cured with radiation therapy, and can be cured with effective chemotherapy even when the disease is widely spread and systemic symptoms are present. Patients with indolent non-Hodgkin's lymphomas (NHL) very rarely have localized disease that can be cured with radiation therapy, have a very high response rate to chemotherapy, but can rarely be cured. Finally, a minority of patients with aggressive NHL have localized disease that can be cured with radiation therapy, but even patients with extensive disease can potentially be cured with aggressive chemotherapy.

When making a treatment decision for a patient with lymphoma, the physician has available the same three treatment modalities used in the treatment of all malignancies. These include surgery (a local mode of therapy), radiation therapy (also a treatment modality that is generally applied locally but on occasion can be a systemic form of therapy), and chemotherapy (almost always used as a systemic therapy). Because of the natural history of the lymphomas, surgery is an effective mode of therapy only in the occasional aggressive NHL that begins at an extranodal site and is discovered before dissemination. Radiotherapy is a highly effective treatment modality for localized (Stage I and sometimes Stage II) lymphomas and total body radiotherapy is an effective systemic treatment in the disseminated, indolent NHLs. However, the majority of patients with lymphomas have disseminated disease (Hodgkin's disease approximately 50% of the time, aggressive NHL approximately 70% of the time, and indolent NHL

Table 1
Major Clinical Subgroups of Lymphoma

1. Hodgkin's disease
2. Aggressive non-Hodgkin's lymphomas
   a. diffuse histiocytic
   b. diffuse undifferentiated
   c. diffuse mixed
   d. diffuse poorly differentiated lymphocytic
   e. nodular histiocytic
   f. lymphoblastic lymphoma
3. Indolent non-Hodgkin's lymphomas
   a. diffuse well-differentiated lymphocytic
   b. nodular poorly differentiated lymphocytic
   c. nodular mixed

approximately 90% of the time) and are best treated with chemotherapy.

With the development of the first active chemotherapy drugs in the late 1940s, it quickly became apparent that the lymphomas were among the most responsive diseases. Tumorous masses were observed to decrease in size and patients' performance status often increased with their use, but considerable toxicity and inability to produce cures with the use of single agents soon tempered enthusiasm. A "standard" approach was to administer chemotherapeutic agents only to patients with advanced disease when other potentially curative modalities such as radiotherapy had failed to cure the patient or seemed unlikely to succeed. To minimize toxicity, the agents were used one at a time in sequence. In the mid 1960s, the concept of combination chemotherapy was developed and applied in the treatment of Hodgkin's disease. The successful application of combination chemotherapy depends upon the presence of several active agents with different modes of action and nonoverlapping toxicities. When these drugs are administered at doses close to that appropriate for the use of each drug as a single agent, the chances for emergence of a resistant tumor cell population are decreased and thus the chances for cure improved. The studies at the National Cancer Institute in the treatment of Hodgkin's disease with meclorethamine, vincristine (Oncovin), procarbazine, and prednisone (MOPP) exemplified this approach. It soon became apparent that a significant proportion of patients so treated achieved complete remission and did not relapse on prolonged follow-up. In the early 1970s it became apparent that long-term disease-free survival with combination chemotherapy could also be achieved in the aggressive NHLs. Unfortunately, similar success has not been achieved with the use of combination chemotherapy in the treatment of the indolent NHLs.

The goal of treatment today in patients with Hodgkin's disease and aggressive NHL, irrespective of stage, is cure. Except for the occasional patient with localized disease, cure with currently available therapy in the indolent NHL is unusual. The ability to cure patients with disseminated lymphoma is dependent on the development of combinations of active chemotherapeutic agents and appropriate strategies for their use. One key point in this regard has been the recognition of the importance of "complete remission" as a goal of therapy. A "complete remission" in this context means the absence of disease after completion of therapy and a careful "restaging" evaluation. In general, this means any previously abnormal physical findings, laboratory evaluations, radiological studies, and biopsies have been repeated and have normalized. Patients who achieve a complete remission after therapy for Hodgkin's disease and the aggressive NHL will be cured in the majority of cases. Unfortunately, most patients with indolent NHL will eventually relapse despite achieving documented complete remission.

When making a therapeutic decision in patients with a lymphoma, there are many disease, patient, and treatment variables that should be considered. Perhaps the most important single factor to be taken into consideration is the histological subtype of the lymphoma. Hodgkin's disease and the aggressive NHLs are generally rapidly fatal and always require therapy as soon after diagnosis as is practical. The indolent NHLs have a prolonged natural history that allows considerable flexibility in the timing of initiating therapy. In some asymptomatic patients with indolent NHL therapy can be delayed indefinitely. No matter what the pathological subtype of lymphoma, the rate of progression of the disease in the individual patient, the occurrence of unpleasant symptoms, and the involvement of vital organs by the disease, need to be taken into account in the treatment decision. For example, a newly diagnosed patient with an indolent NHL with rapidly enlarging lymph nodes, fever, night sweats, and ureteral compression by retroperitoneal tumor would require urgent treatment despite the "favorable" histological subtype. Patient factors also deserve consideration in the therapeutic decision. It is obvious that one might approach a 90-year-old patient with organic brain syndrome residing in a nursing home differently from a 25-year-old mother of two young children. In addition to age, the patient's general medical condition and ability to tolerate therapy need to be taken into consideration. For example, a patient with congestive heart failure would be a poor candidate to receive adriamycin. Even if from every other point of view the patient with an indolent NHL would require no initial therapy, treatment may need to be initiated because of the patient's inability to tolerate delay once they have been told they have a malignant disease. Failure to recognize this latter point will drive some patients to seek care elsewhere.

When therapy is to be initiated, the morbidity and the potential benefit (i.e., is cure possible?) of the various treatments available need to be taken into consideration. The chemotherapeutic agents useful in the management of lymphomas frequently have unpleasant short-term and long-term side effects. Early untoward reactions to the drugs include nausea, vomiting, alopecia, and sepsis. Potential long-term complications include sterility, altered sexual function, and treatment-induced second neoplasms. When cure is the goal of therapy, especially in younger patients, it is relatively easy to decide to accept these risks. However, in a patient who is not disabled, and in whom cure is not an achievable goal, these potential treatment complications might outweigh the potential gains.

Finally, many patients will not be cured with the currently available therapies. How to manage these patients after it becomes apparent that cure is not possible, given that the relative merits of currently available salvage therapies are not always clear, can present difficult clinical decisions.

The remainder of this chapter will deal separately with each of the three major groups of lymphomas, answering a series of questions relevant to the major decisions that need to be made in managing these patients. The questions are: (1) Are there active agents? (2) Are combinations of drugs better than single agents? (3) Is chemotherapy ever the treatment for localized disease? (4) Is there an effective salvage therapy for patients who fail primary therapy? (5) What are the major treatment-related complications? and (6) What is the best chemotherapy available today?

Are There Active Single Agents?

A definite, clear-cut definition for response to chemotherapeutic agents is a prerequisite for the intelligent use of these drugs. The development of a generally agreed upon definition for response was one of the key steps in the advancement of the discipline of medical oncology. A response is intended to designate clear-cut evidence that the drug in question killed cancer cells and to avoid counting as responses variations due to observer differences or minor fluctuations in the size of tumors unrelated to the treatment. An objective response to a chemotherapeutic drug is said to exist when measurable tumor has decreased by one-half of its surface area (usually the product of the two greatest diameters of the tumor) for a defined period of time (usually 1 or 2 months). A special type of response is a "complete response." This denotes complete disappearance of all signs of the tumor after discontinuing therapy and reevaluation of the patient. Any response less than complete is generally referred to as a partial response. It is important to note that response refers to decrease in the size of the tumor and has nothing to do with improvement in the clinical status of the patient. It is entirely possible for a patient to be more ill because of toxicity of the therapy, even though an objective response occurred. It is also possible for a patient to be improved clinically because of decreased pain secondary to a minor shrinkage of tumor that would not fit the criteria for an objective response.

It is important when interpreting a report of therapy of lymphoma or any other malignancy with drugs that the definitions of response used by the authors be clearly stated and carefully considered. It is also important to note that the previous exposures of a particular tumor to chemotherapy will affect the chances for response to subsequent therapy. For this reason, a patient undergoing salvage therapy with a new drug in the 1980s would, all other things being equal, have a lesser chance to respond than a similar patient in a similar clinical situation in the 1960s. A patient in the 1980s will have been treated with more "standard" agents, on the average, before being offered new, experimental drugs. For all these reasons, it is difficult to be precise when comparing single drug response rates tested in different patients at different times. In the paragraphs below I have tried to identify as "active" a drug capable of causing 20% objective responses. However, it is difficult to compare the relative effectiveness of different single agents beyond identifying them as active.

Hodgkin's Disease

Table 2 lists the active drugs from the major classes of chemotherapeutic agents for the treatment of Hodgkin's disease. As can be seen, there are a great number of active agents and the level of activity in some cases is quite high. Hodgkin's disease is one of the few neo-

Table 2
Active Drugs in Hodgkin's Disease

Class	*Drug*
Alkylating agents	Mechlorethamine
	Cyclophosphamide
	Chlorambucil
	Thiotepa
Antibiotics	Adriamycin
	Bleomycin
Vinca alkaloids	Vincristine
	Vinblastine
Nitrosoureas	CCNU
	BCNU
Miscellaneous	Procarbazine
	DTIC
	VP-16

plasms where single agents are occasionally able to induce complete responses. It is possible, by utilizing single agents in sequence, to control Hodgkin's disease in some patients for extended periods of time. Nevertheless, cure cannot be achieved with this approach.

Aggressive Non-Hodgkin's Lymphomas

As can be seen in Table 3, there are also a number of active agents in the aggressive NHLs. However, the number of agents are fewer than in Hodgkin's disease and the level of activity is generally less. Complete remission with use of single agents in these tumors is unusual.

The Indolent Non-Hodgkin's Lymphomas

Table 4 lists the activity of the major classes of chemotherapeutic agents in the indolent NHLs. As can be seen, there are a number of active agents. The level of activity is generally greater than seen in the aggressive NHLs. In addition, complete responses are possible with prolonged use of single agents.

Initial management in the indolent non-Hodgkin's lymphomas frequently involves the use of chlorambucil or cyclophosphamide as a single agent. The treatment is generally given orally, in a dose that the marrow will tolerate for prolonged periods of time (i.e., chlor-

Table 3
Active Drugs in Aggressive Non-Hodgkin's Lymphomas

Class	*Drug*
Alkylating agents	Cyclophosphamide
	Mechlorethamine
Antibiotics	Adriamycin
	Bleomycin
Vinca alkaloids	Vincristine
	Vinblastine
Antimetabolites	Cytarabine
	Methotrexate
Nitrosoureas	BCNU
Miscellaneous	Procarbazine
	Prednisone
	VP-16

ambucil 2–8 mg daily, and cyclophosphamide 100–200 mg daily). Blood counts are monitored regularly to guard against severe myelosuppression. When either of these drugs is utilized in this manner for prolonged periods of time (i.e., up to 1 year or even longer) a complete response rate of 60–70% can be achieved in nodular, poorly differentiated lymphocytic NHL and the overall response rate is even higher. Comparable results are possible in diffuse well-differentiated lymphocytic NHL, but the response rate tends to be lower in the

Table 4
Active Drugs in Indolent Non-Hodgkin's Lymphomas

Class	*Drug*
Alkylating agents	Cyclophosphamide
	Chlorambucil
	Mechlorethamine
	Melphalan
Antibiotics	Adriamycin
	Bleomycin
Vinca alkaloids	Vincristine
	Vinblastine
Nitrosoureas	BCNU
Miscellaneous	Prednisone
	DTIC
	VP-16
	VM-26

nodular mixed NHL and the remissions tend to be of shorter duration. Unfortunately, although complete response can be achieved in greater than one-half the patients, and the median duration of complete responses is several years, almost all patients eventually relapse.

Are Combinations of Drugs Better Than Single Agents?

Certainly one major advance in the use of chemotherapeutic agents was the development of the principles of combination chemotherapy. In most diseases, where a number of highly active drugs are available and can be safely combined to produce a high percentage of complete remissions, some of the patients will be cured. Unfortunately, as will be seen below, this cannot always be achieved.

Hodgkin's Disease

The first attempts at combination chemotherapy in the treatment of Hodgkin's disease took place in the early and mid-1960s. The MOPP regimen that was developed during this time at the National Cancer Institute is one of the prototype combination chemotherapy regimens (see Table 5). This regimen, or slight modifications of it, has now been used in multiple treatment trials in Hodgkin's disease. Early in its use it quickly became apparent that total response rates of approximately 90% and complete response rates of 60–80% could be achieved. Most trials have used a minimum of six cycles of MOPP delivered at approximately monthly intervals and treated patients for at least

Table 5
The MOPP Regimen for Hodgkin's Disease*

Drug	*Dose*
Mechlorethamine	6 mg/m^2 IV days 1 and 8
Oncovin (vincristine)	1.4 mg/m^2 (maximum dose 2 mg) IV days 1 and 8
Procarbazine	100 mg/m^2 PO days 1–14
Prednisone	40 mg/m^2 PO days 1–14 (often given only in cycles 1 and 4)

*Repeated at 28-day intervals for six cycles and at least two cycles post disappearance of clinically apparent disease.

two cycles after a clinical complete remission was achieved. Patients who were then carefully restaged and found to be without evidence of disease have remained free of Hodgkin's disease 50–80% of the time. When relapses do occur, they are usually soon after discontinuing therapy. The median time to relapse is approximately 18 months after discontinuing therapy, and relapse after 4 years off therapy is extremely unusual. Early in the treatment of Hodgkin's disease with MOPP, there was a serious question that patients who achieved a complete remission might benefit from maintenance chemotherapy. This has been studied in controlled clinical trials and, although relapse is delayed in patients receiving maintenance chemotherapy, the ultimate cure rate is not changed. Because maintenance treatment is at best a nuisance and is associated with some risk without long-term benefit, maintenance therapy in Hodgkin's disease has largely been abandoned.

It quickly became apparent that MOPP was a significant advance in the treatment of Hodgkin's disease over the use of single agents. This has been studied and confirmed in a controlled clinical trial comparing MOPP to mechlorethamine alone. However, whether some other combination chemotherapy regimen would be superior to MOPP for the treatment of Hodgkin's disease is a point for ongoing study.

Aggressive Non-Hodgkin's Lymphomas

As noted above, the use of single agents in the treatment of the aggressive NHLs was largely unsuccessful. Complete remissions were unusual and the median survival in the largest group of patients (i.e., those with diffuse histiocytic lymphoma) was in the order of 1 year. Survival beyond 2 years was unusual. A series of patients with these aggressive lymphomas were treated with the MOPP regimen (or the C-MOPP regimen where cyclophosphamide is substituted for mechlorethamine) at the National Cancer Institute in the 1960s and early 1970s. It was found that 43% of these patients achieved a complete remission and the majority of these patients did not relapse on prolonged follow-up. This significant improvement in the treatment of the aggressive NHLs has subsequently been confirmed with other chemotherapy regimens. The most popular and most successful regimens have incorporated adriamycin. Perhaps the most frequently used of these has been the CHOP regimen utilizing cyclophosphamide, adriamycin, vincristine, and prednisone (see Table 6). Utilizing this regimen, complete remissions can be achieved in more than 50% of

Table 6
The CHOP Regimen for Aggressive Non-Hodgkin's Lymphomas*

Drug	*Dose*
Cyclophosphamide	750 mg/m^2 IV day 1
Hydroxyldaunomycin (adriamycin)	50 mg/m^2 IV day 1
Oncovin (vincristine)	1.4 mg/m^2 (maximum dose 2 mg) IV day 1
Prednisone	100 mg PO days 1–5

*Repeated at 21–28 day intervals for six cycles and at least two cycles post disappearance of clinically apparent disease.

the patients and approximately two-thirds of these patients will not relapse on prolonged follow-up when complete remission is documented by careful restaging evaluation.

Indolent Non-Hodgkin's Lymphomas

The use of combination chemotherapy was approached with enthusiasm in this very responsive group of diseases. The most popular combination regimens, developed in the late 1960s and early 1970s, were combinations of cyclophosphamide, vincristine, and prednisone, variously abbreviated COP or CVP. Complete response rates of 50–75% were achieved although at a higher price in toxicity than was seen with the use of single agents. Unfortunately, unlike the situation found in Hodgkin's disease and the aggressive NHLs, the complete remissions in these patients were not found to be durable. Median complete remission durations as long as 5 years were frequently found. However, the pattern of a few early relapses and the subsequent flattening of the remission duration curve seen in the more aggressive lymphomas were not found in these patients. The remission duration curves tend to show a steady rate of decline that continues progressively between 5 and 10 years of follow-up and suggest that none, or very few, of these patients are cured. This discouraging situation has been approached in several ways. One possibility that has been tested is that more intensive therapy might achieve cure. As a general rule, the early combination regimens for indolent NHL used fewer drugs and were less intense than regimens used for the aggressive non-Hodgkin's lymphomas. However, the use of very aggressive combination regimens, including the CHOP regimen, has not improved the results.

The importance of intensity of therapy in the indolent NHLs has been studied in a randomized clinical trial at Stanford University Medical Center. Patients received either daily therapy with a single alkylating agent (i.e., either chlorambucil or cyclophosphamide), combination chemotherapy with CVP, or combination chemotherapy with CVP combined with total lymphoid irradiation (TLI). The complete remission rates varied from 65% for the single agent therapy, to 70% for CVP and TLI, to 83% for CVP alone. These differences were not statistically significant. However, the time to achieve a complete remission was much longer with single agent therapy. The median durations of the complete remissions were essentially identical and were approximately 4 years. There was no survival advantage with any of the therapies and 70% of the patients remained alive at 7 years. Thus, there was no advantage of combination chemotherapy over single agent chemotherapy in this clinical trial.

The one type of indolent NHL in which there has been a serious argument presented that combination chemotherapy is superior to single agent chemotherapy *and* potentially curative is the nodular mixed lymphocytic-histiocytic subgroup. In a series of patients treated at the National Cancer Institute with the C-MOPP regimen, more than half were reported to have long-term disease-free survival with a remission duration curve demonstrating a plateau suggestive of cure. The same result has not been found in several other clinical trials and remains a point for debate.

In summary, at the present time it is impossible to document definitely improved results with the use of combination chemotherapy over single agent therapy in the indolent NHLs. Whether or not these patients can be cured with chemotherapy is unclear. However, it is worthwhile to remember that when treating a group of patients with a median age well in excess of 60 years, median complete remission durations of 4 to 5 years and median survivals of 7 to 10 years can be very useful results. Many elderly patients will die of other causes before they die of an indolent non-Hodgkin's lymphoma. It should also be remembered that when these diseases occur in young patients, their initial, comparatively benign course is deceptive and these diseases will eventually lead to the death of the patient.

Is Chemotherapy Ever the Therapy for Localized Disease?

When chemotherapeutic agents are demonstrated to be able to cure patients with bulky, advanced disease who have systemic symptoms, the possibility should be considered that the same approach might be more effective for patients with minimal disease. However, the effectiveness of radiation therapy for patients with localized lymphomas has slowed the study of chemotherapy for localized disease. As will be noted below, a few studies have suggested that chemotherapy is a highly effective treatment for patients with localized lymphomas. However, the longer duration of therapy with drugs compared with radiation and the more severe immediate side effects of chemotherapy have left radiation the treatment of choice for localized (Stage I) lymphomas in the eyes of most oncologists in this country.

Hodgkin's Disease

The results of therapy with MOPP for patients with asymptomatic (i.e., lacking fevers, night sweats, and weight loss) Hodgkin's disease has been extraordinary. Five-year disease-free survivals in excess of 90% have been achieved in more than one series. With these results in patients with extensive (Stage III or Stage IV) disease, it is reasonable to assume that even better results might be achieved in patients with less bulky (Stage I or Stage II) disease. However, there is very little clinical experience in the treatment of localized Hodgkin's disease with drugs. This is largely due to the proven effectiveness of radiotherapy in the treatment of these patients. Several years ago, a group of physicians treating Hodgkin's disease in Uganda did have occasion to treat a series of patients with localized Hodgkin's disease with MOPP. This came about due to the absence of radiotherapy equipment in that country. Eleven patients with Stage I and II Hodgkin's disease were treated and all achieved a complete remission. Approximately 70% of these patients were long-term disease-free survivors. These results suggest that combination chemotherapy is probably an effective treatment for patients with asymptomatic, localized Hodgkin's disease. However, the disadvantages of chemotherapy when compared with radiotherapy for localized disease make it unlikely that chemotherapy will become the standard treatment for this disease in the United States.

Aggressive Non-Hodgkin's Lymphomas

Radiotherapy is an effective mode of treatment for patients with carefully staged Stage I aggressive NHL. Cure in these patients will be in excess of 80–90%. However, the results are not nearly as good in the patients with Stage II aggressive NHL, and cures in most series are well below 50%. For this reason, many oncologists would now routinely treat patients with Stage II aggressive NHL with drugs.

The effectiveness of combination chemotherapy in the treatment of patients with asymptomatic but disseminated aggressive NHL suggests that this same treatment might be highly effective in patients with considerably less disease. Two series of patients, treated at the University of Arizona and at M.D. Anderson Hospital in Houston, Texas, suggest that this is in fact the case. In 44 patients with Stage I and Stage II aggressive NHL treated at these institutions with only chemotherapy, 41 (93%) achieved a complete remission. Thirty-six of the 41 complete responders (88%) had durable complete remissions at the time the series were reported. These results are comparable to what can be achieved with radiation therapy in Stage I aggressive NHL and are definitely superior to that achieved with radiation therapy in Stage II non-Hodgkin's lymphomas. The prolonged time to complete chemotherapy and the occurrence of more severe early side effects will still make radiation therapy the treatment of choice for many oncologists in patients with carefully staged Stage I aggressive non-Hodgkin's lymphomas.

Indolent Non-Hodgkin's Lymphomas

Localized disease in the indolent NHL is unusual. With careful staging, 80–90% of patients will have extensive (Stage III or Stage IV) disease and only a few patients will have Stage I disease. However, for these few patients it appears that radiation therapy is potentially curative. Because the potential for cure with chemotherapy in the indolent NHL is uncertain, I believe it is difficult to defend treatment of patients with definitely localized disease with drugs. With the very high likelihood of disseminated disease, some authors feel that aggressive staging is not appropriate and patients should be treated immediately with chemotherapy. However, when no contraindications to the various staging procedures exist, I believe it is worthwhile to identify the few patients who will have localized, indolent NHL so that curative radiotherapy can be applied.

Is There an Effective Salvage Therapy Available for Patients Who Fail Primary Treatment?

The majority of patients who develop lymphomas extensive enough to be treated with drugs will not achieve initial remission or will eventually relapse and become candidates for salvage therapy. These will include approximately half the patients treated for Hodgkin's disease with chemotherapy, over half the patients with aggressive NHL treated with chemotherapy, and almost all patients with indolent NHL treated initially with chemotherapy. As will be seen below, our ability to salvage these patients leaves much to be desired. One of the important areas for future study in the treatment of lymphomas is to identify patients unlikely to be successfully treated with currently standard regimens so they can receive alternative therapies.

Hodgkin's Disease

One of the areas of continuing controversy in the treatment of Hodgkin's disease is the best way to manage patients who fail initial drug therapy. It has become clear that all patients who fail initial drug treatment do not have the same prognosis. Patients should be divided into those initially refractory to MOPP or another combination regimen, those who fail shortly after achieving a complete remission (i.e., in less than 1 year), and patients who have late relapses after achieving an initial complete remission. Patients who are initially refractory to drug therapy in Hodgkin's disease have a very poor outlook. These patients are unlikely to achieve long-term disease-free survival with further drug therapy. Patients who relapse shortly after achieving a complete remission are similar to those initially refractory to treatment. Neither of these groups of patients should be retreated with their previous treatment regimen. Unlike the first two groups, patients who relapse after achieving complete remissions of a year or longer appear to be frequently sensitive to retreatment with their initial regimen—at least when the initial regimen was MOPP. Of 15 patients in the National Cancer Institute series who relapsed more than a year after achieving complete remission with MOPP, 14 (93%) achieved a second complete remission on retreatment with MOPP. The outlook for patients in this latter group is considerably better than for patients with no initial remission or rapid relapse after discontinuing therapy.

Because of the large number of active agents in Hodgkin's disease, it is possible to develop non-cross-resistant regimens with multiple drugs. A number of these have been developed and have been used to treat patients who fail MOPP or an alternate regimen (Table 7). Most of these treatment trials have been with MOPP failures, but there are also ABVD (adriamycin, bleomycin, vinblastine, dacarbazine) failures treated with MOPP. Although a fair number of complete remissions can be achieved, the majority of these remissions are not durable and the long-term disease-free survival rate with salvage therapy ranges from 0–25% in various series. It is apparent that patients who fail initial combination chemotherapy for Hodgkin's disease have a very poor outlook.

Because of the results detailed above, many oncologists would treat patients failing one combination chemotherapy regimen, and certainly after failing two combination chemotherapy regimens, utilizing single agents with palliative intent. The large number of active agents available and the occasional patient with slowly progressive disease can make this approach successful at achieving an improved quality of survival in many patients. It is important to remember that single agent chemotherapy is much less likely to have serious side effects than combination chemotherapy. The most useful drugs to use in this setting, in my experience, tend to be vinblastine on a weekly basis or procarbazine on a daily oral basis. However, "shopping" through the available drugs trying to minimize toxicity and maximize life quality is often necessary for the best result.

Table 7
Salvage Chemotherapy Regimens in Previously Treated Hodgkin's Disease

Regimen	*Complete Response Rate*	*Long-Term Disease-Free Survivors*
ABVD (adriamycin, bleomycin, vinblastine, DTIC)	59%	23%
B-DOPA (bleomycin, DTIC, vincristine, prednisone, adriamycin)	60%	0%
Adriamycin + CCNU	50%	0%
CVB (CCNU, vinblastine, bleomycin)	50%	0%
ABDIC (adriamycin, bleomycin, DTIC, CCNU, prednisone)	34%	17%

It is also important to remember that occasionally radiotherapy can be very helpful in this setting. At times the least toxic maneuver to achieve palliation of symptoms in patients with advanced Hodgkin's disease is radiation of symptomatic lesions.

Aggressive Non-Hodgkin's Lymphomas

As a general rule, the outlook for patients with aggressive NHL is poorer than for Hodgkin's disease. This rule extends to the benefits of salvage therapy. This may partly be related to the older age of patients with NHL but is undoubtedly also related to the very aggressive nature and lower drug responsiveness of these diseases. There have been a number of combination chemotherapy regimens used to rescue patients who fail initial chemotherapy. When patients with aggressive NHL are treated initially with CVP, an occasional patient will achieve long-term disease-free survival when subsequently treated with an adriamycin-based four-drug regimen (e.g., CHOP). The value of further combination drug therapy in patients who fail more modern aggressive chemotherapy regimens is less clear. The same general rules apply for the aggressive NHL as for Hodgkin's disease. That is, the more refractory the disease, such as in patients who fail initial therapy or fail rapidly after discontinuing therapy, and the more treatment regimens failed all indicate a poorer prognosis with salvage therapy.

Multiple combination chemotherapy regimens have been tried as salvage treatment in the aggressive NHL (see Table 8). As can be seen,

Table 8
Salvage Chemotherapy Regimens in Previously Treated Aggressive Non-Hodgkin's Lymphoma

Regimen	*Complete Response Rate*	*Long-Term Disease-Free Survivors*
PVB (cisplatin, vinblastine, bleomycin)	27%	—
IMVP-16 (ifosfamide, methotrexate, VP-16)	38%	12%
High dose methotrexate	17%	—
V-Plat (VM-26, cisplatin, prednisone)	17%	—

these regimens have complete response rates varying from 0–30% with the majority of the complete responders subsequently relapsing. The chances for long-term disease-free survival after salvage chemotherapy is poor, with no series showing a cure rate as high as 20%. These patients should be considered candidates for innovative new therapies, such as marrow transplantation.

The success with single agent salvage chemotherapy described above for Hodgkin's disease cannot be achieved in the aggressive NHLs. These patients are extremely unlikely to achieve a complete response with single agent chemotherapy, and the duration of partial responses tends to be brief. Patients with aggressive NHL who fail initial, potentially curative combination chemotherapy form a particularly refractory subgroup with a very poor outlook.

Indolent Non-Hodgkin's Lymphomas

To a significant degree, the story of treating indolent NHL with drugs is a story about salvage therapy. Almost all patients who achieve initial complete remissions will eventually relapse and require salvage therapy. Fortunately, these patients are much more likely to respond to further chemotherapy than patients with aggressive NHL. Patients with indolent NHL who have failed to achieve an initial complete remission with chemotherapy, however, have a poorer outlook with salvage therapy than patients who relapse after achieving an initial complete remission. As a general rule, treatment of patients who relapse after a prolonged complete remission should be reinstitution of the initial chemotherapy regimen, unless some contraindication exists. Patients who are refractory to their initial regimen or relapsed promptly after its discontinuance should generally receive alternative treatment regimens. Because of the number of active drugs in these lymphomas, a considerable variety of treatment options is available. It is important to remember that the judicious use of radiotherapy to relieve symptomatic lesions or eliminate unattractive, bulky adenopathy can often be particularly useful.

One important reason for treatment failure in the indolent NHLs that should always be kept in mind is transformation to an aggressive histological variety of lymphoma. This usually means transformation of the diffuse well-differentiated lymphocytic NHL, nodular poorly differentiated lymphocytic NHL, or nodular mixed lymphocytic-histiocytic NHL, to a diffuse histiocytic lymphoma. Histological transformation occurs in more than half of patients with prolonged survival. In patients with new or recurrent lymphadenopathy, particularly if associated with new symptoms, a biopsy should be performed whenever possible. Patients who transform from an indolent NHL to diffuse histiocytic lymphoma form a particularly refractory subgroup for further therapy. Long-term disease-free survival is unusual and the chance for a useful response to chemotherapy is less than in patients who continue with an indolent histological subtype.

What Are the Important Complications of Chemotherapy in the Lymphomas?

There are two broad categories of complications related to chemotherapy for lymphomas that can each be subdivided. The first includes the immediate effects of treatment appearing during therapy. These can be further subdivided into "nuisance" side effects that are unpleasant but not dangerous and the more serious immediate side effects. The most common "nuisance" side effects that occur in the treatment of the lymphomas with drugs include nausea, vomiting, alopecia, and distal extremity parasthesias. Although these are generally not dangerous, they are often the most important aspect of therapy to the patient. Any efforts to reduce the severity or duration of the side effects can have a profound positive effect on the patient's quality of life and allow some patients, who would otherwise refuse to be treated, to continue therapy. The more dangerous immediate side effects relate to the effects of the drugs on various vital organs. By far the most important of these is myelosuppression. Anemia and thrombocytopenia can generally be corrected easily, but infections in the presence of granulocytopenia are a major threat. This problem can be worsened by the immunosuppressive effect of concurrently administered prednisone. Death due to infection is the most important and most frequent fatal side effect of chemotherapy for lymphomas. Other organs, however, can also be damaged. These include the heart, secondary to adriamycin usage, lung disease, secondary to a number of agents, and hepatic dysfunction that can also be caused by more than one agent.

When treatment is initiated for a lymphoma, the threat of the malignancy is the outstanding concern of both the patient and the physician. However, the treatments can lead to delayed, serious side effects that appear long after the lymphoma has disappeared. Delayed, important side effects of the chemotherapy of lymphomas can include loss of fertility, alteration in sexual function that can sometimes lead to divorce, chronic organ dysfunction (congestive heart failure or avascular necrosis of bone), and treatment-related second neoplasms. The most important of the latter is acute nonlymphoblastic leukemia.

Hodgkin's Disease

Unpleasant, immediate side effects from the chemotherapy of Hodgkin's disease are one of the outstanding features of most of the commonly used regimens. Both MOPP and ABVD have a tremendously high incidence of nausea and vomiting, which is frequently very severe. Occasionally patients will refuse to continue therapy because of this problem. Treatment-related alopecia is more frequent with ABVD than with MOPP. Serious immediate side effects seen with both regimens are generally related to the immunosuppressive effects of the treatments. Deaths due to infection have been reported in as many as 11% of patients undergoing treatment for Hodgkin's disease with MOPP.

The delayed side effects of chemotherapy for Hodgkin's disease can be significant. This is particularly so because of the relatively young average age of patients with Hodgkin's disease. When the MOPP regimen is utilized, there is a high incidence of infertility and altered sexual function. The alteration in sexual function generally involves both loss of libido and, in males, impotence. While the frequency of infertility appears lower with ABVD than with MOPP, the effect of ABVD on sexual function has not been so clearly described in the literature. The altered sexual function in young, married patients with Hodgkin's disease may be one of the reasons for the high divorce rate that has been reported in these patients.

The delayed side effect of the treatment of Hodgkin's disease with drugs that has received the most attention has been treatment-related second neoplasms—particularly acute nonlymphoblastic leukemia. The frequency of occurrence of acute nonlymphoblastic leukemia after chemotherapy for Hodgkin's disease seems to be related to the presence of an alkylating agent or procarbazine in the treatment regimen. For this reason, the frequency of acute nonlymphoblastic leukemia after treatment with ABVD has been much less than seen with MOPP. There seems to be a dose response effect for the occurrence of acute leukemia after cytotoxic chemotherapy. Thus, patients who are treated on multiple occasions, or given maintenance chemotherapy, are at a higher risk. The actual frequency of acute nonlymphoblastic leukemia complicating treatment of Hodgkin's disease with MOPP seems to be on the order of 5–10% in patients with prolonged follow-up.

Aggressive Non-Hodgkin's Lymphomas

Most regimens currently used for the treatment of aggressive non-Hodgkin's lymphomas include an alkylating agent, adriamycin, vincristine, and prednisone, with or without other drugs. The anticipated immediate side effects with these agents include nausea and vomiting (occasionally severe), alopecia (which can frequently be decreased by scalp cooling during and immediately following drug infusion), and distal extremity parasthesias. The latter side effect may occur more frequently, or at least be more bothersome, in older patients. Because very intensive drug regimens are usually used to treat patients with aggressive NHL, myelosuppression is frequently severe. This leads to treatment-related early deaths in as many as 10–20% of patients. The frequency of treatment-related early deaths seems to be, at least in part, an age-related phenomenon. It is much more likely in patients over 70 years of age (see Table 9).

The delayed side effects of the treatment of patients with aggressive NHL with drugs are significant. The actual frequency of side effects seen in a series of patients treated at the University of Iowa for diffuse histiocytic lymphoma with CHOP are presented in Table 10. As can be seen, treatment-related second neoplasms were not a major problem. This has also been the experience of others. Occasional patients had persistence of unpleasant, acute side effects of drug treatment. These included treatment-related distal extremity parasthesias, or alopecia, in less than 10% of treated patients. By far the most frequent, unpleasant delayed side effect was alteration in sexual function, seen in 60% of patients who were sexually active at the time of initiation of therapy. Perhaps because of the advanced age of these patients (i.e., median age 65 years), this was not associated with any divorces.

Indolent Non-Hodgkin's Lymphomas

Because of the less intensive regimens generally used to treat the indolent NHL, immediate side effects tend to be less severe. Although occasional patients treated with single agent chemotherapy or the less intensive combinations will be bothered by nausea and vomiting, this is much less a problem than is seen with regimens such as MOPP or CHOP. When single agent chlorambucil therapy is used, treatment is

Table 9
The Effect of Age on Treatment-Related Mortality in Patients with Diffuse Histiocytic Lymphoma Treated with CHOP*

Age Group	*Number of Patients*	*Early Deaths (%)*
33–69 years	55	1 (2%)
70–94 years	20	5 (25%)

*The groups are significantly different, $p < .01$.

usually without unpleasant side effects. However, myelosuppression can still occur and occasional treatment-related deaths due to sepsis will be seen. These will be much less frequent than with the more intensive regimens used to treat the aggressive non-Hodgkin's lymphomas.

The most important delayed treatment-related complication appears to be the occurrence of acute nonlymphoblastic leukemia. This is probably related to the fact that these patients have multiple relapses and undergo multiple treatments over extended periods of time. Treatment-related acute nonlymphoblastic leukemia reached a cumulative rate of 8% after 10 years in patients treated at the National Cancer Institute. Other delayed treatment-related side effects seem to be less frequent in this group of patients—probably also related to the less intense therapies they tend to undergo.

Table 10
Frequency of Possible Late Sequelae to Therapy in a Group of Patients with Diffuse Histiocytic Lymphoma Successfully Treated with CHOP

Side Effect	*Frequency of Occurrence*
Altered sexual function	60%
Low performance status	22%
Persistent paresthesias	17%
Congestive heart failure	17%
Loss of employment	15%
Persistent alopecia	9%
Divorce	0%

What Is the Best Currently Available Chemotherapy for Patients with Advanced Lymphomas?

As is true with most diseases where the available treatment is not entirely satisfactory, there is no consensus as to the exact, best approach. In the paragraphs below, I will outline the most popular approaches, try to identify their advantages and disadvantages, and present what I feel to be a reasonable therapeutic plan.

Hodgkin's Disease

The arguments for the "best" chemotherapy regimen to treat advanced Hodgkin's disease generally fall into three categories. One argument is that the MOPP regimen is the most proven treatment option currently available with the longest follow-up and should be considered standard. Others would argue that there are alternative combination chemotherapy regimens available with similar complete response rates and a decreased incidence of immediate and/or delayed side effects that make them preferable (e.g., ABVD). Still others would argue that combining MOPP and ABVD into one drug regimen, despite the inherent increase in side effects, produces a higher response rate and should thus be the favored treatment approach. Table 11 compares the reported results of therapy of advanced Hodgkin's disease with several treatment regimens exemplifying the best points of the various treatment approaches.

I do not believe that one can be certain that any particular treatment regimen is distinctly superior to the others. All of the regimens produce complete response rates in approximately 70–80% of patients, and the majority of complete responses are durable. As a general rule, all the treatment regimens do less well in patients with B symptoms, patients with extensive extranodal disease (e.g., bone marrow involvement), and in patients over 40 years old. It should be noted that many of the most popular drug regimens for Hodgkin's disease have been used in conjunction with adjuvant radiotherapy to sites of bulky disease. The exact contribution of the radiation to the ultimate cure rate is hard to determine.

At the present time I believe the "standard" therapy for Hodgkin's disease should still be MOPP (see Table 5). In patients who lack systemic symptoms, MOPP is an outstanding treatment regimen with greater than 90% of the patients surviving 5 years after initiating

Table 11
Initial Chemotherapy Regimens for the Treatment of Advanced Hodgkin's Disease

Regimen	*Complete Response Rate*	*Long-Term Disease-Free Survivors*
MOPP (See Table 5)	80%	55%
ABVD (adriamycin, bleomycin, vinblastine, DTIC) + / − Radiotherapy	71%–94%	—
BCVPP (BCNU, cyclophosphamide, vincristine, procarbazine, prednisone)	77%	50%
ChlVPP (chlorambucil, vinblastine, procarbazine, prednisone) + / − Radiotherapy	77%	53%
MOPP/ABVD (alternating)	92%	64%

therapy. The results of treatment in patients with systemic symptoms is considerably poorer and the cure rate is less than 50%. It is this group of patients where the combination of MOPP and ABVD was originally suggested to be a major therapeutic advance. It is too early to tell whether or not this will turn out to be the case. Certainly, at the present time, I do not believe that MOPP-ABVD should supplant MOPP as the standard for all patients with advanced Hodgkin's disease.

Aggressive Non-Hodgkin's Lymphomas

Despite their rapid growth rate and relatively poor outlook, the aggressive NHL can be cured with combination chemotherapy. Although the chances for cure vary with the presence or absence of certain prognostic factors (e.g., lower chance for cure with B symptoms or bone marrow involvement), every patient has a chance for cure and should be approached with that in mind. The optimal drug regimen for the treatment of these patients is not at all clear. All the available treatment regimens have considerable toxicity and fail to cure every patient. At the present time it is impossible to say with confidence that one regimen is clearly superior to the others. The merits of the most popular regimens are discussed in the following paragraphs.

The drug regimens used to treat the aggressive NHL can be considered according to the number of incorporated drugs. The early combination regimens used to treat these tumors incorporated three drugs—usually cyclophosphamide, vincristine, and prednisone. The chance for cure with this approach was approximately 20% in diffuse histiocytic lymphoma (i.e., the prototype for this group of lymphomas) and the toxicity, although significant, was not limiting (see Table 12). The next series of regimens added another drug to the combination of cyclophosphamide, vincristine, and prednisone. The most popular regimens added adriamycin (CHOP) or procarbazine (C-MOPP). These regimens seemed to increase the cure rate to approx-

Table 12
Initial Chemotherapy Regimens for the Treatment of Advanced, Aggressive Non-Hodgkin's Lymphomas

Regimen	*Complete Response Rate*	*Long-Term Disease-Free Survivors*
CVP (cyclophosphamide, vincristine, prednisone)	30–50%	20%
C-MOPP (cyclophosphamide, vincristine, procarbazine, prednisone)	43%	37%
CHOP (see Table 6)	57%	41%
COMLA (cyclophosphamide, vincristine, methotrexate, cytarabine)	55%	37%
COP-BLAM (cyclophosphamide, vincristine, procarbazine, bleomycin, adriamycin, prednisone)	73%	—
M-BACOD (methotrexate, bleomycin, adriamycin, cyclophosphamide, vincristine, dexamethasone)	72%	—
ProMACE-MOPP (prednisone, adriamycin, methotrexate, cyclophosphamide, VP-16, mechlorethamine, vincristine, procarbazine)	74%	—

imately 40%, but with a corresponding increase in toxicity. Another popular four-drug regimen was the COMLA regimen that included cyclophosphamide, vincristine, methotrexate, and cytosine-arabinoside. This produced results approximately comparable to the other four-drug regimens. The CHOP-BLEO regimen was a five-drug program with bleomycin added to the basic CHOP regimen. This program produced results approximately comparable to those that could be achieved with CHOP with little additional toxicity because of a very low dose of bleomycin.

The next generation of drug regimens in the treatment of these tumors came with the introduction of the six to eight drug regimens COP-BLAM, M-BACOD, and ProMACE-MOPP (Table 12). These regimens offered a definite increase in intensity of therapy and a corresponding increase in toxicity. However, they have also demonstrated an increased complete remission rate and this might be ultimately translated into a higher cure rate (see Table 12). The follow-up of patients treated with these regimens is not equal to that with the earlier generations of treatment regimens and whether or not the ultimate cure rate will be improved, or whether late relapses will occur, remains to be seen.

Because aggressive NHLs are rapidly fatal diseases for which we do not yet have perfect treatment regimens (or anything even approaching perfect), I believe these patients are best treated in clinical trials trying to identify improved regimens. However, if participation in a clinical trial is not an option, I believe the following would be a reasonable approach. Patients who lack systemic symptoms, whose disease is confined to lymph nodes, and who lack bone marrow involvement or bulky abdominal masses, have a considerably better outlook than patients with the opposite characteristics. These patients respond more favorably to less intense therapy and for these patients I believe the CHOP regimen (Table 6) is still a reasonable treatment option. Patients who have systemic symptoms, who have disease in the bone marrow, who have bulky abdominal or mediastinal masses, or who have diffuse histiocytic lymphoma after transformation from a previously treated indolent non-Hodgkin's lymphoma, have a poor outlook when treated with CHOP. I believe these patients should be treated with one of the newer, more intensive regimens, such as COP-BLAM.

The "best" treatment for aggressive non-Hodgkin's lymphomas will continue to change over the next several years. Physicians who treat these patients should, if at all possible, participate in clinical trials trying to identify better treatment regimens and must keep up with the advances that will occur in this area.

Indolent Non-Hodgkin's Lymphomas

Treatment regimens that are currently popular for patients with advanced, indolent NHL include observation, single agent chemotherapy, combination chemotherapy, and total body irradiation. In various clinical circumstances, excellent arguments can be made for the use of any of these approaches.

Because of the prolonged natural history and the absence of systemic symptoms in the majority of patients, some patients with indolent NHL can be followed safely without therapy. To be a candidate for this approach, the patient must first of all be satisfied not taking any treatment, should not have unpleasant symptoms from the disease, and must have no immediate life-threatening manifestations of the disease such as ureteral obstruction by large retroperitoneal nodes. When a patient meets these criteria, observation without treatment is a reasonable approach.

Most patients will not, for one reason or another, be candidates for observation without therapy. There is no definite best treatment for them. None of the treatment options available are definitely curative in patients with advanced, indolent NHL and all of the treatment options available have some shortcomings. The simplest approach is chlorambucil, 6 mg orally daily with dose adjustments to keep the white blood cell and platelet counts in a safe range. Despite the potential problems of myelosuppression and the late risk of leukemia, this is an extremely easy approach. Treatment has to be over an extended period of time and it is not unusual to take as long as a year to achieve a complete remission. However, survival with this approach is as good as with any other treatment option.

Combination chemotherapy in the indolent, advanced NHL yields a faster response and quicker complete responses, but is not associated with improved survival. Increasing intensity of therapy yields an increased frequency of side effects but no definite improvement in treatment outcome. Combination regimens of cyclophosphamide or chlorambucil with or without vincristine, and with or without prednisone are the most popular. Whenever life-threatening manifestations of the lymphoma necessitate a prompt response, combination chemotherapy should be the initial treatment. No matter what the combination chemotherapy regimen or other type of treatment that is chosen as the initial therapy, it is important that treatment be continued until the patient achieves a complete remission. A theme common to almost every treatment trial in these diseases is that once therapy has been undertaken, achieving a complete remission is associated with a superior survival.

Table 13
Initial Treatment Regimens for Advanced, Indolent Non-Hodgkin's Lymphomas

Regimen	*Complete Response Rate*	*5-Year Survival*
Single agent chlorambucil or cyclophosphamide	65%	80%
CVP (cyclophosphamide, vincristine, prednisone)	83%	75%
CVP + total nodal radiotherapy	70%	70%
Total body radiotherapy	85%	70%

Table 13 gives the results with the various treatment options that have been utilized in the indolent NHLs. It is apparent that no particular treatment approach is definitely superior to another. The treatment chosen for a particular patient should take into account all the clinical parameters in an attempt to eliminate symptoms, optimize survival, and avoid unnecessary unpleasant side effects.

Selected Reading

Hodgkin's Disease:

DeVita, V.T., Hellman, S.: Hodgkin's disease and the non-Hodgkin's lymphomas, in DeVita, V.T., Hellman, S., Rosenberg, S.A. (eds.): *Cancer: Principles and Practice of Oncology*. Philadelphia, J.B. Lippincott Co., 1982, pp. 1331–1401.

DeVita, V.T., Simon, R.M., Hubbard, S.M., et al.: Curability of advanced Hodgkin's disease with chemotherapy. *Ann. Intern. Med.* 92:587–595, 1980.

Armando, S., Bonadonna, G., Bonfante, V., et al.: Alternating drug combinations in the treatment of advanced Hodgkin's disease. *N. Engl. J. Med.* 306:770–5, 1982.

Glick, J.H., Barnes, J.M., Bakemeier, R.F., et al.: Treatment of advanced Hodgkin's disease: 10-year experience in the Eastern Cooperative Oncology Group. *Cancer Treatment Rep.* 66:855–870, 1982.

Aggressive Non-Hodgkin's Lymphomas:

DeVita, V.T., Hellman, S.: Hodgkin's disease and the non-Hodgkin's lymphomas, in DeVita, V.T., Hellman, S., Rosenberg, S.A. (eds.): *Cancer: Principles and Practice of Oncology*. Philadelphia, J.B. Lippincott Co., 1982, pp. 1331–1401.

Armitage, J.O., Dick, F.R., Corder, M.P., et al.: Predicting therapeutic outcome in patients with diffuse histiocytic lymphoma treated with cyclophosphamide, adriamycin, vincristine and prednisone (CHOP). *Cancer* 50:1695–1702, 1982.

Sweet, D.L., Golomb, H.M., Ultmann, J.E., et al.: Cyclophosphamide, vincristine, methotrexate with leucovorin rescue, and cytarabine (COMLA) combination sequential chemotherapy for advanced diffuse histiocytic lymphoma. *Ann. Intern. Med.* 92:785–790, 1980.

Laurence, J., Coleman, M., Allen, S.L., et al.: Combination chemotherapy of advanced diffuse histiocytic lymphoma with the six-drug COP-BLAM regimen. *Ann. Intern. Med.* 97:190–195, 1982.

Fisher, R.I., DeVita, V.T., Hubbard, S.M., et al.: Diffuse aggressive lymphomas: Increased survival after alternating flexible sequences of ProMACE and MOPP chemotherapy. *Ann. Intern. Med.* 98:304–309, 1983.

Skarin, A.T., Canellos, G.P., Rosenthal, D.S., et al.: Improved prognosis of diffuse histiocytic and undifferentiated lymphoma by use of high dose methotrexate alternating with standard agents (M-BACOD). *J. Clin. Oncol.* 1:91–98, 1983.

Indolent Non-Hodgkin's Lymphomas:

DeVita, V.T., Hellman, S.: Hodgkin's disease and the non-Hodgkin's lymphomas, in DeVita, V.T., Hellman, S., Rosenberg, S.A. (eds.): *Cancer: Principles and Practice of Oncology*. Philadelphia, J.B. Lippincott Co., 1982, pp. 1331–1401.

Portlock, C.S., Rosenberg, S.A., Glatstein, E., et al.: Treatment of advanced non-Hodgkin's lymphomas with favorable histologies: Preliminary results of a prospective trial. *Blood* 47:747–756, 1976.

Portlock, C.S.: Management of the indolent non-Hodgkin's lymphomas. *Semin. Oncol.* 7:292–301, 1980.

Portlock, C.S.: Deferral of initial therapy for advanced indolent lymphomas. *Cancer Treatment Rep.* 66:417–419, 1982.

7

Radiotherapy of Hodgkin's and Non-Hodgkin's Lymphoma

Hamed H. Tewfik, M.D.

Radiation Therapy of Hodgkin's Disease

Radiation therapy is the treatment of choice in Stages I, II, and III-A Hodgkin's disease. Megavoltage equipment should be used; and because of the complex field shaping, planning and shaping of normal tissues, the role of an experienced radiation oncologist is essential.

Optimal radiotherapy can only be given by a radiotherapist experienced in the treatment of Hodgkin's disease with the proper equipment and backup technical support, treatment simulator, and facilities to cut lead blocks to shield normal structures during treatment. Shielding and field shaping are used to protect lungs, spinal cord, larynx, kidneys, gonads, and iliac crest bone marrow.

Modern radiation therapy treatment techniques permit the administration of adequate radiation doses to involved areas including large mediastinal masses and the shielding of noninvolved adjacent tissues such as the lung. While shielding can minimize the risk of certain sequelae such as radiation pneumonitis, the potential exists for improper alignment of lung shields which can lead to inappropriate shielding of the supraclavicular or axillary nodes and can thereby decrease the dose of radiation to these areas. Similarly, an inappropriate gap between the radiation ports can lead to overlap resulting in damage of the over-treated area. For example, this may lead to spinal cord injury or radiation myelitis.

Radiotherapy is the treatment of choice for early stage disease, combination chemotherapy is the primary treatment for advanced-stage disease or with parenchymal organ involvement, and a combination of the two is recommended for patients when apparently localized disease is associated with adverse prognostic factors such as bulky disease (large mediastinal mass or very large nodes) or B symptoms.

The major features of modern radiation therapy for Hodgkin's disease are the following: (1) utilization of megavoltage radiation beams having the capability of treatment to large volumes; (2) high dose of radiation to the tumor volume; (3) tailoring of radiation portals to conform to the patient's anatomy in the treatment position.

The advantages of the linear accelerator with an energy from 4–10 MeV over the cobalt unit for the treatment of a patient with Hodgkin's disease are the following: (1) large volumes can be treated relatively quickly and usually at shorter distances than with a cobalt unit; (2) the linear accelerator is associated with less scatter radiation outside the main radiation volume and this may determine subsequent hematological tolerance to salvage chemotherapy in those patients who fail radiation treatment.

The initial plan of treatment for Hodgkin's disease, as well as non-Hodgkin's lymphoma, is very critical in determining the outcome. Careful initial staging is important since appropriate radiation therapy can be curative if treatment fields encompass all disease. The use of megavoltage radiation therapy and extended fields to include contiguous, but clinically uninvolved, nodal sites is essential in obtaining high cure rates.

Sequential irradiation consists of delivering radiation therapy to lymph nodal areas on both sides of the diaphragm. Total nodal irradiation (TNI) sequentially irradiates a mantle field above the diaphragm followed by an inverted "Y" below the diaphragm. Sometimes total nodal irradiation is called total lymphoid irradiation (TLI).

Subtotal nodal irradiation (STNI) (or long-tailed mantle) refers to a mantle followed by a paraaortic splenic pedicle field and has become the arrangement most widely used in laparotomy-negative Stage I-A and II-A patients. The advantage of the long-tailed mantle arrangement is that it avoids radiation therapy to the pelvis and pelvic bone marrow and the amount of scatter radiation to the gonads is minimal.

Radiation Therapy With Curative Intent

In radiation therapy with curative intent, radiation doses in tumorocidal range should be delivered. Also, the use of a minimal number of large fields should be carefully shaped and aligned to encompass all the major lymph node chains. It is now well documented that the recurrence rate in each treated field is inversely related to dose and becomes negligibly low at total radiation doses of approximately 4000–4400 cGy (rad) delivered in 4½–5½ weeks.

At each junction line between adjacent radiation fields a serious potential hazard exists of overlapping of fields with corresponding overdosage and significantly increased probability of tissue injury, or of an excessive gap with underdosage to affected lymph nodes lying near the plane of the junction. This consideration has led to the development of sophisticated techniques for megavoltage beam shaping which made it possible to carry out total lymphoid radiotherapy with a minimal number of extremely large fields carefully shaped, designed, and aligned.

While radiation therapy is the treatment of choice for Stages I-A and II-A disease, the best therapy for Stages I-B and II-B disease has not been yet established. High relapse rates using radiation therapy alone in Stage II-B has suggested that combined treatment (radiation and chemotherapy) may be the optimal treatment. However, the small number of Stages I-B and II-B patients available for a controlled study makes it difficult to have definitive answers.

Clinical studies have suggested that the optimal dose for local control of Hodgkin's disease in the grossly involved lymph nodes in the irradiated field is approximately 4500 cGy (rad) in 5–6 weeks.

Nodal sites on the same side of the diaphragm as the clinically apparent disease receive 4000 cGy followed by a 500 cGy boost to the involved areas only. The dose per fraction of treatment is 150–200 cGy. A total dose of 3500 cGy is adequate for nodal sites on the clinically uninvolved side of the diaphragm.

Treatment to the paraaortic nodes and splenic pedicle area is recommended even in laparotomy-negative supradiaphragmatic Stages I-A and II-A patients since microscopic disease below the diaphragm cannot be dependably detected even at surgery.

Patients with Stage I or II Hodgkin's disease who are treated with mantle radiotherapy and who fail the treatment are most likely to fail in one or two patterns: (1) Subdiaphragmatic extension, most commonly seen in patients who present with cervical adenopathy, especially when left-sided involvement has been noted. (2) Extension into the pulmonary parenchyma and pleura, a type of failure most frequently seen in patients who have large mediastinal and hilar involvement. The subdiaphragmatic extension of Hodgkin's disease has almost been eliminated in Stage I and II patients by the use of prophylactic subdiaphragmatic field irradiation. The term "prophylactic" is a misnomer. The administration of such a field cannot prevent the development of Hodgkin's disease in a site at which there is no disease. Rather, the administration of such a field is preventive on the statistical basis of microscopic involvement of specific sites that may have eluded the most extensive modern diagnostic techniques, even including surgery. Although there are no conclusive data to demonstrate that the concept of preventive irradiation can be extended to the pulmonary parenchyma as well, there are data which suggest that a low dose of irradiation to the entire lung, when hilar and/or parenchymal lung disease is known to be present, can decrease the probability of subsequent parenchymal and/or pleural involvement in such patients. Radiation therapy alone may be inadequate for patients who have extranodal extension to the lung or mediastinal masses larger than one-third the diameter of the chest.

The principals of treatment for Stage I and II Hodgkin's disease depends upon the thesis of contiguous lymphatic spread. The results of modern radiotherapy show that local failure within the radiation field is a relatively infrequent event; most patients who fail radiation therapy fail because of extension beyond the radiation field.

Clinical and pathological Stage I and II-A supradiaphragmatic disease without large mediastinal masses should be treated with a mantle and paraaortic field radiation, except for those with lymphocyte depletion histology, which should receive at least total nodal irradiation and, in some centers, chemotherapy as well. Even when systemic symptoms are present in Stage II disease, clear benefit, survival, and relapse-free survival have not been achieved with combined modality treatment. Consideration of radiotherapy alone for a patient with clinical Stage II-B disease is probably a major indication for a staging laparotomy, since its findings should influence a definitive treatment plan for such a patient.

The majority of patients with Stage I and II-A disease have little or no mediastinal involvement; the relapse free-survival is 92% and overall survival is 97% using the technique that spares the pelvis from irradiation. Although Stage II-A patients without large mediastinal mass have cure rates exceeding 90% with radiation therapy alone, the presence of a large mediastinal mass reduces the chance of cure with radiation alone to approximately 50%. This suggests that these patients should receive combined modality therapy—radiation therapy and chemotherapy. Administration of a portion of the planned chemotherapy prior to radiation therapy offers the potential advantage of shrinking the tumor mass, thus allowing reduction in the size of radiation therapy ports and less toxicity.

Clinical and pathological Stage I and II-A disease with large mediastinal masses is actually a subgroup of Stage I and II-A patients who have a higher likelihood for relapse, especially when those masses are greater than one-third of the total chest diameter. Patients relapsed both within the initial treatment area as well as in adjacent untreated lymph nodes and extranodal relapse is primarily in the lung. These patients are more likely to recur even at involved sites separate from the mediastinum. Despite the high failure rate, subsequent treatment of these patients with chemotherapy has resulted in excellent survival. It should be noted that irradiation of these extensive mediastinal lesions causes additional problems as it may require irradiation of a large volume of the lung or heart. Such patients are also anesthesia risks, so laparotomy in this group carries an additional hazard. A variety of techniques have been used in an attempt to reduce pulmonary complications. Whole lung irradiation has been given to patients with hilar lymph node involvement using tolerable doses or transmission blocks that allow only a portion of the dose to reach the lungs.

An alternative is to use radiation as in the other Stage I and II patients, but to use techniques of dividing the mantle irradiation into two courses to allow the mass to shrink and thus reduce the area irradiated in the second course. Radiation therapy has been given to large pulmonary masses to a dose of 1500 cGy (rad) over 2 weeks, then stopped for 2–3 weeks to allow time for the mass to shrink. The radiation is then continued using smaller ports. The major advantage of the reduced dose, when the mediastinal component is large, is to decrease the amount of radiation to the lungs which are known to have quite limited tolerance to radiation when a large volume of parenchyma is included. After approximately 2 weeks off treatment, a second course with much larger lung blocks to protect more lung tissue can usually be planned. If the mediastinal mass is extremely massive and slow to shrink, a second split-off treatment may be used at approximately 3000 rad. Such treatment will be associated with an approximate 50% chance of failure. Most of these patients, however, can be salvaged with subsequent chemotherapy.

A treatment option appears to be initial combination chemotherapy with radiation to areas of previous bulky disease (mediastinum). Such a treatment modality means that, in patients presenting initially with a large mediastinal mass, laparotomy is not indicated since it will not alter therapy and does carry an anesthesia risk. Full dose chemotherapy should be given with the radiation volume restricted; the total dose of radiation required under such circumstances is uncertain.

The use of combined modality treatment in Stages I and II patients is controversial. The use of chemotherapy in addition to radiation is favored by some when B symptoms are present. When mediastinal masses are too large to be treated with radiation, many recommend chemotherapy for two or three cycles before the initiation of radiation therapy, but it should be noted that the use of four cycles of MOPP (mustard, Oncovin, procarbazine, prednisone) chemotherapy prior to radiation is considered excessively toxic.

The subdiaphragmatic portion of radiation therapy for Hodgkin's disease will cover the paraaortic nodes, splenic hilum, spleen (if not removed), and often iliac and inguinal nodes. The need to encompass the iliac and inguinal nodes is uncertain when nodular sclerosing Hodgkin's disease is present, particularly when there are no systemic symptoms and when there are geographically suspicious nodes that are specifically biopsied at the time of surgical staging and found to be negative. If systemic symptoms are present, the iliac and inguinal nodes are usually treated by total nodal irradiation. The preventive dose is usually reduced to 3500 cGy (rad). Documentation of splenic involvement implies a major risk of hepatic involvement, even when a liver biopsy is negative. Such splenic involvement dictates that the liver be treated on a preventive basis either by MOPP chemotherapy in combination with radiotherapy or by incorporating the entire liver in the radiation portal to a modest dose of about 2500 cGy (rad). Higher doses are risky because of the possibility of radiation-induced hepatic injury. Since microscopic hepatic involvement in this condition is a statistical probability, the lower dose is appropriate.

One should be careful of the preventive field radiation in children because it will arrest bone growth, especially when the child is less than 13 years of age.

There is uniform support for the concept that combination chemotherapy is the standard treatment of Stages III-B, IV-A, and IV-B Hodgkin's disease. Controversy surrounds the proper management of Stage III Hodgkin's disease. The results in Stage III-B with radiotherapy alone are so poor that such treatment is probably inappropriate. Therapy of Stage III Hodgkin's disease represents an area of controversy because radiation therapy alone, chemotherapy alone and combined modality therapy have been alternatively advocated.

It has also been shown that patients who relapse after receiving chemotherapy almost always relapse at previously major involved sites, especially bulky sites suggesting that chemotherapy alone may not be capable to erradicate disease. Combined treatment has therefore been recommended for patients with advanced Hodgkin's disease.

Anatomical substages of Stage III have been suggested to be based on the extent of abdominal nodal disease and can be divided into two anatomical substages. Substage III_1 is defined as involvement above and below the diaphragm, with abdominal disease limited to the spleen, splenic hilar, celiac, and porta hepatic nodes. Substage III_2 defines involvement of paraaortic, mesenteric, iliac, or inguinal nodes, with or without involvement of upper abdominal sites. A recent report of 130 patients who underwent staging laparotomy prior to receiving radiation therapy, or radiation therapy plus combination chemotherapy, evaluated the importance of Stage III substages.

In Stage III-A_1, radiation therapy resulted in an 8-year relapse-free survival of 60%; combined modality therapy was associated with a significantly better relapse-free survival of 92%. However, in Stage III-A_1 patients relapsing after radiation therapy, salvage chemotherapy was highly successful and therefore the overall survival was statistically equivalent for the two treatment groups. So in Stage III-A_1 patients, radiation therapy appears to be adequate and there is no evidence that combined modality therapy improves the clinical results. In contrast to that, radiation therapy alone was inadequate for Stage III-A_2. At eight years, relapse-free survival using radiation therapy alone was only 19% in contrast to an 84% relapse-free survival achieved with radiation therapy plus combination chemotherapy. The salvage chemotherapy was less effective in these patients, probably because most of the relapses occurred at visceral sites. In view of this, overall survival in the radiation therapy group was only 41%, much less than the 84% obtained in patients receiving combined modality therapy. This is a strong indicator that patients with Stage III-A_2 should be treated with either combined modality or chemotherapy alone. In view of the above evidence, pathological stage (PS) III-A patients are best subdivided into favorable III-A_1 and unfavorable III-A_2.

It is recommended that combination total nodal irradiation (TNI) and MOPP should be avoided because of the high risk of secondary malignancies and fatal infections. Therefore, PS III-A_1 patients are treated with TNI. If the patient fails this treatment, then combination chemotherapy should be used. An alternative for clinical Stage III-A and III-B patients is treatment with combination chemotherapy, either alone or with combination chemotherapy and limited volume irradiation to sites of bulky disease (for example, patients with nodular sclerosing Hodgkin's disease). In Stage III-A, over 50% of patients treated with radiation therapy will relapse; the majority of these can be salvaged by subsequent combination of chemotherapy.

Treatment of Stage II-B and III-B Hodgkin's disease with TNI alone can result long-term relapse-free survival in approximately 30% of patients. For pathological Stage II-B disease, irradiation alone may have the same results as combined treatment modality. Since TNI alone in Stage III-B Hodgkin's disease has produced cures in less than 10% of patients, either chemotherapy or combined radiation/chemotherapy appears to be the best modality for this stage. Although adequate information is not unavailable to assist in choosing between the modalities, these therapeutic approaches can produce durable remissions and probably cures in about 60–70% of patients. So, for Stage III-B disease, radiation therapy alone is unsatisfactory treatment. Stage IV-A and IV-B patients should be treated with combination chemotherapy.

Consolidation irradiation delivering relatively low dose radiation (1500–2000 cGy) to sites of initial involvement in patients with advanced disease (Stage III-B or Stage IV) who achieve complete remission on chemotherapy improves the 5-year survival.

Hodgkin's disease treatment may be divided into three areas to be irradiated (Figure 1): the mantle, the paraaortic area, and the pelvis. The mantle technique has been well described by the Stanford group. The lymph nodes of the neck, axillae, mediastinum, and occipital and preauricular lymph nodes are treated in continuity as one contiguous treatment area. The mantle field irradiates a large volume of normal tissues and therefore extreme care must be taken to limit unnecessary normal tissue irradiation while at the same time assuring adequate irradiation and coverage of the tumor volume. This requires careful evaluation and treatment planning, simulation, dosimetry calculation, measurement, and custom-made blocks for shielding.

Clinical stage (CS) and pathological Stage (PS) I and II-A supradiaphragmatic disease without large mediastinal masses should be treated with mantle and paraaortic field radiation, except for those with lymphocyte depletion histology, who should receive at least TNI and, in some centers, chemotherapy as well. Management of CS and PS I and II-A disease with large mediastinal masses has already been discussed. Subdiaphragmatic CS and PS I and II-A disease should be treated with paraaortic and pelvic irradiation for pelvic or inguinal presentation and with TNI for paraaortic involvement. PS II-B disease can be treated with subtotal nodal irradiation. It does not seem that combined modality therapy should be used in such patients unless they have very large mediastinal masses. CS II-B disease should be treated with TNI.

The treatment of the paraaortic nodes and pelvis are frequently done together, as described by the Stanford group. It is the experience

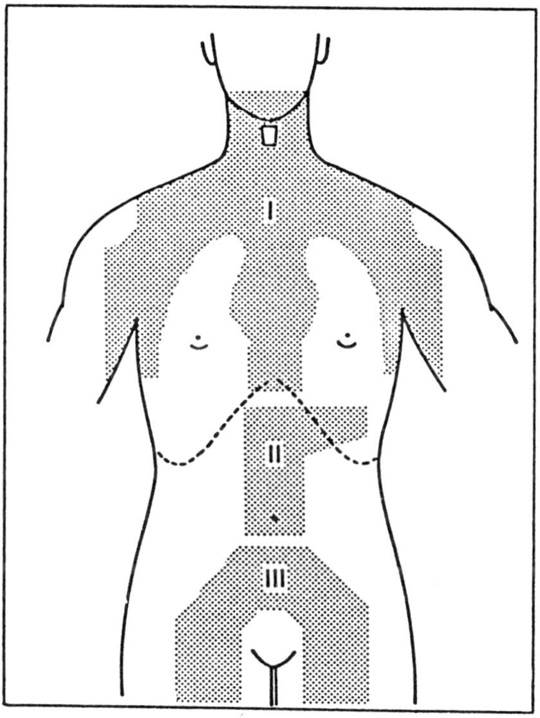

Figure 1: This diagram illustrates radiation fields employed in Hodgkin's disease: I = mantle; II = paraaortic–splenic; III = pelvic. I + II = subtotal nodal irradiation (STNI or long tailed mantle); I + II + III = total nodal irradiation (TNI).

of many other radiation oncologists that this treatment is better tolerated when divided into a paraaortic field and a separate pelvic field. The paraaortic field must be wide enough to include the paraaortic lymph nodes demonstrated by lymphangiography.

Laparotomy is only of value if the information obtained might alter therapy. It allows removal of the spleen and the placement of radioopaque clips on the splenic pedicle, so that the radiation therapy field may be tailored accurately to this volume, also minimizing radiation to the left kidney. Consideration for the pelvic field includes treatment of the lymph nodes with as little radiation as possible to important sacral and pelvic bone marrow. The marrow irradiated may be greatly reduced by careful blocking. Adequate covering of the inguinal and femoral lymph nodes must be assured and the testes should be shielded. In females, a central block can be placed when the ovaries have been fixed either in front of or behind the uterus at laparotomy.

It is generally recommended that local tumor masses receive treatment of a minimum dose of 4000–4400 cGy in 4½–5½ weeks, while apparently uninvolved areas to be treated for subclinical disease appear to be adequately controlled with doses of 3500 cGy in 3½ weeks.

Exceptions to these general recommendations must be applied to very young children who may have a greater risk of infectious complications after splenectomy. Radiation therapy in the dose ranges used in Hodgkin's disease results in significant retardation of growth in the treated area. This area must be limited and care taken to attempt symmetrical irradiation in order to limit the deformity produced as a consequence of asymmetric bone growth.

Controversy still surrounds the proper management of Stage III-A Hodgkin's disease. The British National Lymphoma Investigation compared TNI with MOPP combination chemotherapy in 117 patients with Stage III-A Hodgkin's disease, of whom 81 had staging laparotomy. There was a significant difference in complete response rates, 95% versus 74%, favoring TNI. The relapse-free survival favored those patients receiving TNI who achieved a complete response. The overall survival, however, was identical in the two limbs. The significance of splenic involvement alone in Stage III-A_s versus splenic plus nodal involvement Stage III-A_{sn} was studied by Levi and Wiernik. Their data showed that patients with Stage III-A_s treated with extended field radiotherapy had a relapse-free survival comparable with Stage II-A Hodgkin's disease and a better survival rate than Stage III-A_{s+n+}. Furthermore, limited radiotherapy plus MOPP improved the relapse-free survival of patients with Stage III-A_{s+n+} disease.

Dresser et al. suggested that patients with PS III-A Hodgkin's disease be separated into those with upper abdominal involvement (III_1) and those with lower abdominal involvement (III_2). A retrospective analysis showed the 5-year survival rate of Stage III-A (93%) exceeded that of Stage III-A_2 (57%). Likewise, patients with Stage III-A_2 benefited from combined chemotherapy and radiotherapy. In a multi-institutional collaborative retrospective study, Golomb et al. found further evidence to support the subgrouping of Stage III-A disease. Hoppe et al. on the other hand have separated their patients into subgroups III-A_1, III-A_2 and found that there is no significant difference in freedom from relapse, or survival, among patients treated with TNI alone. They did, however, show that the extent of splenic involvement in patients with Stage III-A_2 Hodgkin's disease (five or more gross splenic nodules) had an adverse influence on freedom from relapse.

Combined modality therapy (chemotherapy and radiotherapy) at the onset in the management of Hodgkin's disease is to be used only in those instances in which there has been a proven survival advantage. The information reported by Golomb et al. showed such a survival advantage for the combined modality in Stage III-A_2. On the other hand, Portlock et al. showed with salvage treatment of initial radiotherapy relapses, using radiotherapy and/or chemotherapy, patients with Stage III-A disease achieve a sustained second response resulting in a survival comparable with the group that received combined modality at the onset.

It seems that TNI is favored for the management of Stage III-A disease, with chemotherapy reserved for those who relapse. This method of management avoids exposing half the patients with Stage III-A disease, i.e., those with III_2, to the risk of acute leukemia which increases with intensity of treatment. A change of this approach may require a randomized prospective controlled clinical trial with stratification into Stages III-A_1 and III-A_2.

In the only randomized trial in which MOPP plus TNI was compared with MOPP alone in Stage IV disease, there was no significant difference in disease-free or overall survival at 7 years. The data of Hoppe and associates for Stages III-B and III-B_s disease reveal a 79% disease-free survival at 3½ years using alternating chemotherapy and irradiation. The most recent data from Bonadona et al. show a 95% and 93% 4-year disease-free survival rate for MOPP plus radiotherapy versus ABVD (Adriamycin, bleomycin, vinblastine, DTIC) plus radiotherapy, respectively. It would appear that the hypothesis first suggested by Frei and associates, that patients receiving varying doses of irradiation to areas of major bulk disease, either following or alternating with chemotherapy, has improved the relapse-free survival rate. Implementation of this in practice must await additional controlled trials.

In summary, radiotherapy is the mainstay of treatment for early stage disease and a combination is required for patients with bulky disease (large mediastinal mass) and/or generalized abdominal nodal involvement.

Results of Treatment

The most important single parameter is survival. Nevertheless, freedom from relapse is also important in that it gives an estimate of cure with any given treatment. Optimally, the 5-year disease-free survival rate (and presumably cure) is 95% in Stage I-A and 85% in Stage II-A. When appropriate doses are given only to sites of involvement in Stages I and II-A Hodgkin's disease after extensive staging that may include laparotomy, the long-term disease-free survival rate is only about 35%. If TNI including the mantle, paraaortic nodes, splenic hilum, and ileofemoral nodes are treated with such doses, the long-term disease-free rates range from 80–90% for Stages I and II-A Hodgkin's disease. When systemic symptoms are present, involved field irradiation alone is considered inappropriate because of the very high probability of relapse. TNI for Stage II-B Hodgkin's disease is associated with long-term disease-free rates of approximately 80%.

TNI may be far more extensive than the intended irradiation of subclinical contiguous disease in Stages I and II-A disease. That is why, for supradiaphragmatic disease, pelvic irradiation may be eliminated. This is important as it will greatly reduce the amount of bone marrow irradiated and would reduce the dose to the gonads. This approach for supradiaphragmatic Stages I and II-A patients is the treatment recommended at the Joint Center for Radiotherapy, Harvard University, and has yielded relapse-free and overall survival rates for Stage I of 91% and 95%, respectively, and for Stage II-A, 79% and 92%, respectively, with only 2% pelvic nodal recurrence. This seems to indicate that the pelvis can be spared from irradiation while patients still derive the value of extended field irradiation. This technique should be adopted in laparotomy-staged patients from whom the spleen has been removed. This approach also avoids the high risk of sterility associated with pelvic irradiation in men and the necessity for oophoropexy in women, while demonstrating that the untreated pelvis was at low risk for recurrence in patients with pathologically staged supradiaphragmatic Hodgkin's disease. Among these early stage patients was a subgroup identified as high risk for relapse. These were patients with initial large mediastinal adenopathy who characteristically relapsed extranodally in the lung or at nodal sites above the diaphragm. As a result of successful chemotherapy with nitrogen mustard, vincristine, procarbazine, and prednisone (MOPP) at the time of recurrence, similar survival rates have been reported for these patients regardless of whether initial radiation therapy alone (with MOPP reserved for treatment failure) or combined modality treatment was used.

According to Hellman et al., in Stage I-A treated with radiotherapy alone survival at 5 years is 100%, while freedom from relapse at 5 years is 97%. For Stage II-A, radiotherapy alone resulted in 93% and 80% survival rates, respectively. For Stage II-B, radiotherapy with MOPP survival rates were 86% and 82%, respectively. According to Rosenberg et al., survival rates for Stages I-A and II-A with radiotherapy alone were 84% and 71%, respectively; for Stages I-A and

II-A radiotherapy with MOPP, 95% and 87%, respectively; for Stage II-B radiotherapy alone, 89% and 79%, respectively; and for Stage II-B radiotherapy with MOPP, 87% and 84%, respectively. In patients with Stage III-A Hodgkin's disease staged by laparotomy and treated with TNI, the 5-year survival and relapse-free survival rates are 65% and 46%, respectively.

Patients with PS I-A or II-A Hodgkin's disease have an excellent relapse-free and overall survival when treated with radiation therapy alone. Treatment with mantle and paraaortic irradiation allows sparing of the pelvic bone marrow and potential preservation of fertility. There have been only 2.4% pelvic nodal failures in patients who have received mantle and paraaortic irradiation, so in some patients there may be a role for lesser irradiation, especially when the initial disease is limited to high neck nodes. Very young or elderly patients with limited Hodgkin's disease might be the most likely candidates for lesser field irradiation.

Infradiaphragmatic Hodgkin's disease with inguinal or femoral adenopathy has a prognosis similar to that for supradiaphragmatic disease.

Pathologically Staged I-B and II-B Hodgkin's Disease

PS I-B and II-B Hodgkin's disease occurs less frequently than similarly staged I-A and II-A disease. One report has randomized Stage I-B and II-B Hodgkin's patients to treatment with either initial TNI alone or with combined TNI and MOPP chemotherapy. Patients treated with TNI had an actuarial 89% survival rate at 8 years compared to an 87% actuarial survival rate with TNI and MOPP.

There is a paucity of information available on the treatment of Stage II-B Hodgkin's disease, as the number of patients from any one center is small. In Stage II-B patients who were treated with TNI, a 70% 5-year survival rate has been reported; the treatment results with extended field irradiation were not as satisfactory, presumably because of the presence of occult disease below the diaphragm. In a randomized study from Stanford, PS II-B Hodgkin's disease patients had similar relapse-free and overall survival rates whether they were treated with TNI alone or with initial combined modality therapy. Patients had a relapse-free survival rate at 8 years of 79% with radiation therapy alone and of 84% with combined treatment. However, overall survival rates were 89% and 87%, respectively. Patients with Stage II-B Hodgkin's disease reported in this study have an 89% survival rate at 8 years regardless of whether initial radiation therapy alone or combined modality therapy was used. The majority, however, were treated with mantle and paraaortic irradiation with sparing of the pelvic lymph nodes.

The Influence of Histology Upon Relapse-Free and Subsequent Survival of Patients

Nodular sclerosing and lymphocyte predominant histology appear to confirm a more favorable prognosis in patients with Stages I-A or II-A Hodgkin's disease, although the influence of histology upon relapse-free and overall survival of patients with early stage Hodgkin's disease is somewhat controversial. A large proportion of the patients that have been analyzed were not surgically staged and results may simply reflect a low probability that CS I and II patients with nodular sclerosing or lymphocyte predominant histology have occult disease below the diaphragm. These differences have not been seen in studies in which surgical staging has been routinely performed. Nodular sclerosis has a better prognosis in Stages I-A and II-A but not in Stage II-B. The patients with nodular sclerosing histology appeared to fail with relapses in the lung, pleura, or nodal sites above the diaphragm and patients with mixed cellularity histology have a much higher relapse rate in liver, bone, and bone marrow.

Patients With Large Mediastinal Masses

There appears to be a subgroup of patients with large mediastinal adenopathy who are at high risk for relapse. These relapses characteristically occur extranodally in the lung or pleura, as mediastinal recurrences within the treated area, in the margin of the treated field, and at other lymph node sites above the diaphragm. The judicious use of whole lung irradiation and perhaps a higher total dose administered to the mediastinum may help prevent some of these recurrences, but this may significantly increase the risk of complications. Studies have reported no difference in overall survival of patients with large mediastinal adenopathy treated initially with combined modality therapy when compared with radiation therapy alone, MOPP being reserved for relapse.

There are other problems with patients with mediastinal masses. Anesthesia, especially extubation, is more difficult with such masses and thus the mass may require initial irradiation to reduce its size.

Furthermore, the radiation fields required may be very large, increasing the risk of pneumonitis and pericarditis, or causing extended interruptions in treatment that might increase the possibility of local failure. The proper treatment for patients with large mediastinal masses is rather uncertain. In patients with lesser or no mediastinal disease, it is unlikely that the addition of MOPP chemotherapy can significantly improve upon the 88% actuarial freedom from first relapse reported for Stages I-A and II-A. When good technical radiation therapy is available, the acute morbidity and the substantial risk of sterility in both males and females following administration of MOPP chemotherapy can be avoided with early stage patients.

Complications of Treatment

These are related to techniques employed, dose administered, and the irradiated area.

Acute Reactions (Or Acute Side Effects)

When irradiation is delivered to the mantle field, the following acute reactions may occur: dryness of the mouth, loss of taste, dysphagia, dry or moist desquamation (particularly around the neck and axillae), some tanning of the skin, epilation (particularly in the occipital area), nausea, vomiting, apathy, and lassitude. Dysphagia usually resolves within a week to 10 days. Most patients find that weakness, tiredness, lassitude, and apathy start to improve a week after treatment is completed. The skin changes disappear uneventfully. The dryness of the mouth and loss of taste may take as long as 3 months to disappear, and in some patients a thick, tenacious saliva will be present for as long as 6 months. When epilation occurs, the hair grows back in about 3 months.

Complications related to paraaortic field irradiation in Hodgkin's disease are quite uncommon and gastrointestinal complications are a rarity. When treating the paraaortic nodal area below the diaphragm, a slight to moderate amount of nausea, vomiting, anorexia, lassitude, and diarrhea may occur. Nausea and vomiting disappear shortly after the end of treatment. Appetite returns in about a week and rarely does diarrhea persist longer than that. Pelvic treatment alone may cause persistent thrombocytopenia or leukopenia, but this is quite rare with current modern techniques.

Late Side Effects

The most frequent complications of radiation therapy are associated with mantle irradiation. It is unusual to see complications from the staging laparotomy or from paraaortic treatment. The reported incidence of pericarditis is 1.5%, radiation pneumonitis 3.4–10%, clinical hypothyroidism 3.4%, and mild to moderate xerostomia 2.9%. There is also temporary bone marrow suppression in most patients. A higher rate of radiation pericarditis and pneumonitis have been described in some series; however, this appears to be related to area irradiated, daily fractionation, total treatment time, and total dose. When equally weighted anterior and posterior fields are used and when normal lung can be blocked after 1500 cGy and partly blocked after 2500–3000 cGy, the complication rates are low.

The introduction of a subcarinal lead shield, to protect the midportion of the heart and lower mediastinum to a level 5–6 cm below the carina after a total of approximately 3000 cGy has been delivered, reduces the hazard of radiation carditis and pericarditis. One-third of the patients who receive mediastinal irradiation will develop some laboratory evidence of pericardial and/or cardiac dysfunction that is seldom of any significance. The 3.4% incidence of clinical hypothyroidism is lower than that reported previously. This may be due partially to the use of a laryngeal block at 2000 cGy and a posterior spinal block at 3000 cGy, as practiced by the Stanford group. Many patients are followed with routine thyroid-stimulating hormone (TSH) determinations and, if elevated levels are noted, they receive thyroid supplementation before clinical hypothyroidism develops. Subclinical hypothyroidism detected by an elevation in TSH is common (30–40%) and is treated with thyroxin replacement.

If the pelvis is irradiated, the gonads receive significant doses even when appropriate shielding is used. Permanent aspermia may occur with inguinal field irradiation even with small doses of scattered irradiation when the total dose exceeds 200 cGy. Temporary aspermia or menstrual dysfunction is common, but some recovery usually takes place and pregnancies producing normal offspring may occur. Sterility occurs in most men who are treated with pelvic irradiation, but a few regain their fertility years after treatment. About half of the women who are treated with pelvic irradiation develop amenorrhea which may also reverse with time. Overall, there appears to be 25–50% infertility rate after treatment for Hodgkin's disease. Genetic damage to germ cells is a risk that has been documented. Any of these complications may be aggravated if chemotherapy is combined with irradiation.

The most common neurological complication seen with irradiation is Lhermitte's syndrome, consisting of numbness, tingling, or "electric sensations" which are produced by head flexion. This might occur in 15% of patients treated with mantle fields and is of questionable significance. To date, there has been no indication that this syndrome is in any way related to permanent neurological damage. Lhermitte's sign occurs when the neck is flexed and is appreciated as a sense of electric shock, most commonly in the sacral area, frequently radiating down the back of the legs and occasionally down the arms. It usually appears about 10–12 weeks after completion of treatment and persists for varying periods of time. Findings on neurological examination are entirely normal and there is always spontaneous recovery. Serious spinal cord "transection" can occur when a portion of the cord is included in both the mantle and paraaortic fields. If the overlap is avoided, this complication does not occur at doses of 3600–4000 cGy.

The combination radiation/chemotherapy has been demonstrated to be associated with high risk of acute myelogenous leukemia (about 4% after 7 years) and possibly a higher risk of non-Hodgkin's lymphoma than is associated with either single modality. Despite this, combined modality therapy should not be rejected outright, but should be used only when it offers a substantial improvement in survival that can compensate for the increased leukogenic risk. The risk is far less than that of death from recurrent Hodgkin's disease if less than adequate initial treatment is used.

In reference to long-term complications, development of non-lymphomatous second malignancies is an acknowledged complication in the management of Hodgkin's disease. It is now an established fact that second malignancies in Hodgkin's disease are related to the intensity of treatment. Acute leukemia has been identified as the most common second malignancy. These hematological malignancies occur with increased frequency in patients still in complete remission from their Hodgkin's disease who receive intensive combination chemotherapy and radiotherapy. Data from Stanford indicate that radiotherapy alone has not been associated with increased risk of hematological malignancy. Chemotherapy alone and chemotherapy in combination with radiotherapy clearly have oncogenic potentials. Because of the risk of acute leukemia developing in patients treated for Hodgkin's disease, some of the survival advantage achieved with an aggressive approach may be lost. Thus, the unrestrained use of combined modality management of all patients with Hodgkin's disease is not indicated.

Hodgkin's Disease in Children

Staging laparotomy continues to provide important information in the evaluation of disease in children, although the risk of overwhelming postsplenectomy gram-positive infection remains with a mortality rate in the range of 1–3%.

Radiation Therapy With Palliative Intent

In the great majority of cases, especially in patients with widely disseminated disease, chemotherapy is the treatment of choice for palliation. However, the use of palliative radiation therapy is indicated when the symptoms or signs requiring relief are localized or life-threatening, and may provide prompt and sustained relief. The dose used for palliation should be adjusted to deal with a specific situation; relatively high doses (2500–4000 cGy) in 3–4 weeks are justified for long-term control of distressing or life-threatening manifestations of disease, for example, in cases with superior vena caval obstruction, tracheal compression by mediastinal lymphadenopathy, epidural spinal cord compression, and lytic destruction of vertebrae or weight-bearing skeletal structures. In all other situations, it is recommended to use the smallest dose that will offer substantial relief of the symptom or sign for an interval of time deemed significant in relation to the expected survival of the patient.

Radiation Therapy for Non-Hodgkin's Lymphoma (NHL)

The curative role of radiation therapy in the treatment of NHL is different from that of Hodgkin's disease. While NHL is quite responsive to radiation, only a small population of patients are amenable to cure with local or regional irradiation. In addition to histological variance, the term "non-Hodgkin's lymphoma" includes a variety of clinical situations. For example, lymphoma of the bone, mediastinal lymphoma of childhood and adolescence, and lymphoma in Waldeyer's ring are all quite different and may require different therapeutic approaches. Such approaches range from local field radiation to whole body irradiation and from single agent chemotherapy to aggressive multidrug treatment protocols, as well as a combination of radiation and chemotherapy. In the study of all these approaches it should be remembered that it is extraordinarily easy to make many lymph nodes regress in NHL patients. It is not always clear, however, how frequently one alters the natural history of these diseases with treatment. In order to understand this, one must be careful to distinguish survival from interval to first relapse. The nodular lymphomas may have a more indolent course, with a consistent pattern of relapse and mortality; fixed-time survival such as the commonly used 5-year survival, may in fact be misleading. The survival curves may still continue a downward slope.

Radiation therapy has its major role in the treatment of localized lymphomas. Unfortunately, these Stages I and II nodal lymphomas are quite uncommon presentations in non-Hodgkin's lymphoma. In general, the radiation therapy dose used is 3500 cGy in 3½ weeks for localized NHL, except for the histiocytic variety, in which a dose of 4500–5000 cGy delivered over 5 weeks is suggested.

With the increasing complexity of the potential staging and treatment options available to patients with NHL, an initial multidisciplinary planning conference is advisable for each patient as soon as the histiological diagnosis and clinical stages are complete. The questions that need to be answered are: need for laparotomy, radiation therapy with or without adjunctive chemotherapy or chemotherapy alone, and the sequence of therapy, if they are multimodal. Surgery plays the following roles: (1) The primary role is in establishing diagnosis and an anatomical staging to an appropriate degree. (2) Resection of extranodal and gastrointestinal primaries may be curative, often requiring additional radiation for microscopic residual disease. (3) Splenectomy may be indicated for hypersplenism. (4) Staging laparotomy should be considered only in carefully selected patients, especially in younger patients with apparently localized NHL in whom radiation therapy is to encompass all disease with cure as the goal.

The protean clinical presentations and widely diversified biological behavior patterns of NHL require the treatment recommendations to include considerations of the patient's age and general condition as well as the sites of involvement, stage, and histological subtype. The frequency of widespread extranodal disease initially requires the preservation of adequate marrow function for chemotherapy to be tolerated. Radiation techniques should be designed accordingly. Fields utilized in Hodgkin's disease are often inappropriate for NHL.

Favorable Histology of NHL (NLWD, NLPD, NML, DLWD)

NLWD stands for nodular lymphocytic well-differentiated lymphocytic, NLPD stands for nodular lymphocytic poorly differentiated, NML stands for nodular mixed lymphoma (lymphocytic/histiocytic), and DLWD stands for diffuse lymphocytic well differentiated. In this group, it should be noted that, following extensive sequential staging, only about 15% of patients will have localized disease (Stages I and II).

The Management of Favorable Histology, Non-Hodgkin's Lymphoma

The non-Hodgkin's lymphomas comprise a broad spectrum of lymphoid malignancies with different natural histories, histopathologies, and response to therapy. The diagnosis of favorable histology lymphoma rests on examination of adequate lymph node tissue. Once the diagnosis of a favorable lymphoma has been established, the extent of disease can be assessed utilizing the staging procedures.

There are different treatment options for patients with favorable histology lymphomas: for example, in Stages I and II involved field irradiation or extended field irradiation; in Stages I, II, and III total lymphoid irradiation; and in Stages III and IV combination chemotherapy, whole body irradiation, combined modality therapy, or involved field irradiation. With localized presentations, Stages I or II, radiation therapy is usually employed. Unfortunately, few prospective studies are available to answer the questions of necessary field size and dose for curative intent. Jones et al. reported a median relapse-free survival of approximately 5 years for clinical Stage I patients with NLPD or NML and 3.5 years for Stage II following radiation therapy. All patients received at least 3000–4000 cGy to the involved regions. When analyzed retrospectively, those who received extended field or total lymphoid radiation appeared to have a more prolonged relapse-free survival, although the actuarial curves were not significantly different. However, when tested prospectively in a small group of pathologically staged patients, relapse-free survival was improved for all patients, but no significant differences could be found between involved field treatment and total lymphoid irradiation. The relapse-free survival rate was more than 80% at 5 years. Therefore, local field irradiation therapy appears to be the treatment of choice for patients with localized favorable histology lymphomas who have been pathologically staged. Remembering that the mesenteric lymph nodes and spleen may be involved in as many as 50% of patients with clinical Stage I and II disease, one sees why local radiation therapy yielded poorer relapse-free survival in the retrospective series than in the prospective one.

This group of NHL in localized stages is almost universally nodal. Irradiation is the primary modality of treatment for localized disease. There is no convincing evidence that extended fields are superior to involved fields, but it is prudent to include the immediately adjacent clinically involved nodal group. Doses of 3500–4000 cGy at 150–200 cGy daily are adequate. In some circumstances, even lower doses may be recommended. The 5-year survival for nodular Stage I and II NHL treated by radiation is good, but this disease is indolent and late relapses occur. One-half to two-thirds of Stage I nodular lymphoma patients may be cured by radiation therapy. Radiation has a role in advanced favorable histology NHL.

Whether total lymphoid irradiation is curative in patients with Stage III disease has yet to be determined. Glatstein et al. have reported a retrospective series of 51 patients with nodular lymphoma who were treated with 3500–4000 cGy total lymphoid irradiation. The relapse-free survival rate was 43% at 5 years and 33% at 10 years, with more than 90% of relapses occurring in the first 5 years following therapy. When analyzed according to histology, the relapse-free survival was similar for NLPD and NML. In the majority of patients, initial relapses were confined to non-irradiated nodal sites and the authors suggested that improved results might be achieved by including Waldeyer's ring and the epitrochlear and mesenteric regions with the usual total lymphoid portals. This approach remains to be tested prospectively. Combined chemotherapy and irradiation approaches have been disappointing to date. Neither split-course CVP (cytoxan, vincristine, prednisone) plus TLI or whole body irradiation plus combination chemotherapy, CVP, or C-MOPP has been prospectively proved to be superior to combination chemotherapy alone. The potential benefits of combined modality approaches are just beginning to be tested and a major problem that remains to be solved is how to combine chemotherapy and radiation therapy maximally without compromising the efficacy of either treatment.

If treatment is initially deferred, patients with NLPD or DLWD may not require therapy for several years, while those with NML probably will. The anticipated benefits of therapy in terms of prolonged disease-free survival are greatest for NML.

Management of Unfavorable Histology, Non-Hodgkin's Lymphoma

The unfavorable prognosis non-Hodgkin's lymphomas have been identified as diffuse lymphomas (diffuse poorly differentiated lymphocytic, diffuse histiocytic, diffuse mixed lymphocytic, and histiocytic and undifferentiated lymphomas), as well as nodular histiocytic lymphoma according to the Rappaport classification. The following lymphoma disease categories are considered to have an unfavorable prognosis: (1) nodular histiocytic; (2) diffuse poorly differentiated lymphocytic (DPDL); (3) diffuse histiocytic (DHL); (4) diffuse mixed (DML); and (5) diffuse undifferentiated (DUL).

Following extensive sequential staging, about 40% of these patients will have localized disease. About 25% of these will have an apparently extranodal origin, most commonly gastrointestinal, Waldeyer's ring, thyroid, skin, bone, orbit, breast, or testes. Irradiation is the primary modality of treatment for all localized stages, and adjuvant chemotherapy, particularly for DHL, seems to improve long-term results.

The variability in primary site necessitates an individualized approach to the radiation technique for each patient. There is no clear evidence that extended fields are superior to involved fields, but it is prudent to include the adjacent clinically uninvolved nodal regions. In general, doses of 4500–5000 cGy are advisable, although dose reduction is needed in certain sites to remain within tolerance.

Irradiation for specific sites involved by localized diffuse histology NHL is as follows:

(1) *Waldeyer's ring*. Radiation therapy is given to Waldeyer's ring (nasopharynx, tonsils, base of tongue) to a dose of 4500–5000 cGy with elective irradiation of cervical nodes down to the clavicle (3500–4000 cGy).

(2) *Gastrointestinal tract*. The majority of patients are first treated by surgical resection. Postsurgical irradiation of 1500–2000 cGy is given to the whole abdomen, shielding the kidneys and the liver. The tumor bed is then boosted to 3500 cGy. Massive unresectable abdominal disease requires aggressive chemotherapy with or without consolidation radiation.

(3) *Bone*. Resection or amputation does not improve long-term survival and is contraindicated. Irradiation of the whole bone with a boost to 5000 cGy to the involved segment achieves total control in more than 90% of patients.

(4) *Thyroid gland.* The diagnosis is usually made after thyroidectomy and postoperative irradiation is given to the thyroid bed, both sides of the neck, and to the superior mediastinum.

Multiagent chemotherapy added to radiation therapy, particularly if regional nodes are involved (Stage II-E), may improve long-term results for all presentations of localized diffuse histology NHL. Unfavorable histology NHL of advanced Stage II (massive mediastinal adenopathy, two nodal sites involved, massive abdominal disease) and Stages III and IV, is best managed by aggressive chemotherapy, possibly with radiation for palliation or consolidation. Total lymphoid radiation in Stage III diffuse lymphomas may be of value when used with combined modality treatment of unfavorable histologies. Of patients receiving intensive combination chemotherapy, with half receiving adjuvant irradiation, those who received chemotherapy alone had a 24% 4-year survival rate compared with a 5-year 47% survival rate when combined modality treatment was used. Thus, there appears to be a definite role for combined modality management of advanced unfavorable disease.

Chaffe et al. used total body irradiation (TBI) in the treatment of patients with DPLL. They were able to achieve a 50% 5-year survival, but only 5% were disease-free. They concluded that TBI should be considered a systemic agent and used in combination with chemotherapeutic agents. Young et al. studied randomized comparisons of chemotherapy and radiotherapy (TNI, TBI, or hemi-body) alone or in combination in patients with advanced lymphocytic lymphoma. They achieved a 50% 4-year overall survival with no apparent differences between groups. Harrison et al. treated 46 previously untreated advanced unfavorable histology non-Hodgkin's lymphoma patients with four cycles of CHOP followed by TBI, vincristine, prednisone, and bleomycin, followed by four more cycles of CHOP. Complete remission was achieved in 83%, with 61% of the TBI patients remaining alive and in complete remission for up to 26 months. This is a promising lead in the management of unfavorable histologies.

The vast majority of patients with unfavorable histologies in non-Hodgkin's lymphoma have generalized or advanced disease (Stages III and IV) and are candidates for management with a systemic form of treatment with chemotherapy or radiotherapy. Combination chemotherapy remains the mainstay of treatment in these patients, with radiotherapy a helpful adjunct in selected patients. In general, patient ages greater than 50 years, masses larger than 10 cm in greatest diameter, and bone marrow involvement all represent relatively unfavorable prognostic factors. Miller and Jones and others have recently reviewed the role of radiotherapy in the management of localized diffuse histiocytic lymphoma (DHL), the most common type.

Although Stage III NHL is usually treated with chemotherapy, it may be treated with TNI, or perhaps with comprehensive lymphatic irradiation (CLI). CLI involves sequential irradiation of Waldeyer's ring, mantle, epitrochlear nodes, the whole abdomen, and pelvis to a dose of 2500 cGy. Relapse-free survival beyond 5 years occurs in one-third to two-thirds of patients. Stage IV nodular lymphoma may be treated with low dose fractionated TBI. Fifteen cGy to the total body delivered twice weekly to a total of 150 cGy induces complete remission in 90% with a median duration in excess of 2 years and 3-year disease-free survival in 30–40%. CLI and TBI are hematologically toxic and require careful monitoring, especially of the platelet counts. Close collaboration between radiation therapists and medical oncologists/hematologists is essential.

Studies are being conducted to evaluate the role of consolidation irradiation following chemotherapy in advanced NHL. This involves the use of moderate doses of irradiation (1500–2000 cGy) to initially enlarged nodes.

The classification of non-Hodgkin's lymphoma loses relevance in the pediatric age group, because 95% have diffuse histology and a poor prognosis. Stages III and IV disease are common and leukemic transformation is frequent. Abdominal presentation is the most common form in children (30–40%). Surgery, radiotherapy, and chemotherapy all play an important role in treatment. Burkitt's lymphoma is a high growth fraction tumor that abruptly lyses with chemotherapy. Azotemia, hyperuricemia, hypercalcemia, hyperphosphatemia, hypocalcemia, and lactic acidosis as a result of tumor lysis may lead to sudden death.

Mediastinal lymphoblastic lymphoma occurs predominantly in adolescent boys. Ninety percent of these undergo leukemic transformation and spread to the central nervous system (CNS). Intensive multiple drug therapy is the treatment of choice. CNS prophylaxis is important in high risk situations, such as mediastinal involvement or generalized disease.

The Stanford University group published a report of a series of patients with Stage III non-Hodgkin's lymphoma who were treated with primary high dose (3500 cGy or more) TNI alone. Wide field approaches to the abdomen appear essential in primary radiotherapeutic management of non-Hodgkin's lymphoma because of the frequency of mesenteric involvement, even at presentation. Thus, the techniques for primary radiotherapy in these diseases must be distinguished carefully from those employed in the treatment of Hodgkin's disease. The results of treatment in patients with diffuse or aggressive histology were considered inadequate when compared with the results of combination chemotherapy for diffuse histiocytic lymphoma. Only about 20% of the Stage III patients remained disease-free at 5 years, in contrast to the approximately 40% of patients with diffuse histiocytic lymphoma reported in other series who were cured by combination chemotherapy alone. However, it should be noted that this radiotherapeutic series includes all histologies and was not confined to diffuse histiocytic lymphoma alone. Unequivocal evidence of the curability of diffuse lymphomas, other than histiocytic, by chemotherapy alone is lacking.

The more provocative aspect of the Stanford study was the observation that approximately 35% of the nodular lymphoma patients were relapse-free at 10 years with high dose wide field therapy alone. This compared quite favorably with the results reported with combination chemotherapy alone. More importantly, a small series reported from other institutions appears to confirm the Stanford observations concerning the prolonged disease-free survival seen in patients with Stage III nodular lymphoma who undergo wide field high dose radiotherapy. It should be stressed, however, that in the natural history of patients with nodular lymphoma, 10 years is an insufficient period of time to judge whether or not curative treatment has been delivered.

Combined Modality, Combination Chemotherapy and Radiotherapy, in the Treatment of Advanced Non-Hodgkin's Lymphoma

Given the relatively modest curative results of both primary radiotherapy and primary combination chemotherapy in patients with Stages III and IV advanced non-Hodgkin's lymphoma, it is surprising to see how seldom these two modalities have been combined in curative approaches for these patients. This probably reflects the growing awareness of the potential leukemogenic consequences of combined modality treatment in Hodgkin's disease. It should be noted, however, that chemotherapy usually associated with this uncommon phenomenon includes procarbazine, a compound particularly well known for its potential leukemogenicity in animals. Procarbazine is not commonly employed in the treatment of non-Hodgkin's lymphoma.

TBI has been combined with chemotherapeutic regimens of CVP and compared with CVP alone in a study at the National Cancer Institute. The preliminary results indicated no enhancing responsiveness and no suggestion of benefit in terms of survival or freedom from relapse. The hematological toxicity was more pronounced when the two modalities were combined, as might have been predicted. This study was essentially confined to patients with nodular lymphoma.

In another study from Stanford, the combination high dose (greater than 4000 cGy) total lymphoid irradiation after two cycles of CVP chemotherapy, followed by additional chemotherapy after the completion of irradiation for patients with Stage IV nodular lymphoma was evaluated. The complete response rate, median survival, and actual freedom from relapse did not differ for patients who were randomized to receive CVP alone, or even single agent chemotherapy. It should be noted that the study was limited to Stage IV patients, virtually all of whom had bone marrow involvement.

Radiation is effective in relieving superior vena cava obstruction and alleviating spinal cord compression if given appropriately early to a total of 3000–4000 cGy. Chylous pleural effusions, even in the absence of demonstrable mediastinal adenopathy, may be relieved by irradiation to the mediastinum to a total dose of 2000–3000 cGy. Malignant joint effusions usually respond dramatically to moderate doses of 2000 cGy if no underlying osseous lesions are present. After chemotherapy, persistent and recurrent masses and nodes are also responsive to irradiation and do not appear to exhibit altered radiosensitivity.

Selected Reading

Aisenberg, A.C.: Current concepts in cancer: The staging and treatment of Hodgkin's disease. *Northeast J. Med.* 299:1228–1232, 1978.

Anderson, T., Bender, R.A., Fisher, R.I., et al.: Combination chemotherapy in non-Hodgkin's lymphoma: Results of long-term follow-up. *Cancer Treatment Rep.* 61:1057–1066, 1977.

Andrieu, J.M., Montagnon, B., Bayl-Weisgerber, R., et al.: Chemotherapy-radiotherapy association in Hodgkin's disease, clinical Stages I-A and II-A. *Cancer* 46:2126–2130, 1980.

Arseneau, J.C., Sponzo, R.W., Levin, D.L., et al.: Nonlymphomatous malignant tumors complicating Hodgkin's disease: Possible association with intensive therapy. *New Engl. J. Med.* 287: 1119, 1972.

Bennett, J.M. (Ed.): *Lymphomas I.* Boston, M. Nijhoff, 1981.

Bitron, J.D., Golomb, H.M., Ultmann, G.E., et al.: Non-Hodgkin's lymphoma, poorly differentiated and mixed cell types: Results of sequential staging procedures, response to therapy, and survival of 100 patients. *Cancer* 42:88–95, 1978.

Bitron, J.D., Kinzie, J., Sweet, D.L., et al.: Survival of patients with localized histiocytic lymphoma. *Cancer* 39:342–346, 1977.

Bonadona, G., Lattuada, A., Banfi, A.: Recent trends in the treatment of non-Hodgkin's lymphomas. *Eur. J. Cancer* 12:661–673, 1976.

Bonadona, G., Santoro, A., Valagussa, P., et al.: Improved 5-year survival in advanced Hodgkin's disease by combined modality approach. *Cancer Clinical Trials* 2:217, 1979.

Brereton, H.D., Young, R.C., Longo, D.L., et al.: A comparison between combination chemotherapy and total body irradiation plus combination chemotherapy in non-Hodgkin's lymphoma. *Cancer* 43:2227–2231, 1979.

Brody, R.S., Schottenfeld, D.: Multiple primary cancers in Hodgkin's disease. *Semin. Oncol.* 7:187–201, 1980.

Bush, R.S., Gospodarowicz, M., Sturugeon, J., et al.: Radiation therapy of localized non-Hodgkin's lymphoma. *Cancer Treatment Rep.* 61:1129–1136, 1977.

Carabell, S.C., Chaffey, J.T., Rosenthal, D.S. et al.: Results of total body irradiation in the treatment of advanced non-Hodgkin's lymphomas. *Cancer* 43:994–1000, 1979.

Carmel, R.J., Kaplan, H.S.: Mantle irradiation in Hodgkin's disease: An analysis of technique, tumor eradication, and complications. *Cancer* 37(6):2813–2825, 1976.

Chabner, B.A., Fisher, R.I., Young, R.C., et al.: Staging of non-Hodgkin's lymphoma. *Semin. Oncol.* 7:285–291, 1980.

Chabner, B.A., Johnson, R.E., Young, R.C., et al.: Sequential nonsurgical and surgical staging of non-Hodgkin's lymphoma. *Annals Intern. Med.* 85:149–154, 1976.

Chaffe, J.T., Hellman, S., Rosenthal, D.S., et al.: Total body irradiation in the treatment of lymphocytic lymphoma. *Cancer Treatment Rep.* 61:1149, 1977.

Chilcote, R.R., Baehner, R.L., Hammond, D.: Septicemia and meningitis in children splenectomized for Hodgkin's disease. *New Engl. J. Med.* 295(15):798–800, 1976.

Choi, N.C., Timothy, A.R., et al.: Lose dose fractionated whole body irradiation in the treatment of advanced non-Hodgkin's lymphoma. *Cancer* 43(5): 1636–1642, 1979.

Coleman, C.N., Williams, C.J., Flint, A., et al.: Hematologic neoplasia in patients treated for Hodgkin's disease. *New Engl. J. Med.* 297:1249–1252, 1977.

Coltman, C.A., Jr., Montague, E., Haskins, C., et al.: Chemotherapy (MOPP) and total nodal radiotherapy (TNRT) in pathologic Stage II-B, III-A and B Hodgkin's disease. *Proceedings Am. Assoc. Cancer Res.* 68:216, 1977.

Come, S.E., Chabner, B.A.: Staging in non-Hodgkin's lymphoma: Approach, results and relationship to histopathology. *Clin. Haematol.* 8(3):645–656, 1979.

Cox, J.D.: Central lymphatic irradiation to low dose for advanced nodular lymphoreticular tumors (non-Hodgkin's lymphoma). *Radiology* 126(3):767–772, 1978.

Cox, J.D., Komaki, R., Kun, L.E., et al.: Stage III nodular lymphorecticular tumors (non-Hodgkin's lymphoma), results of central lymphatic irradiation. *Cancer* 47(9):2247–2252, 1981.

DeVita, V., Arseneau, J.C., Sherins, R.J., et al.: Intensive chemotherapy for Hodgkin's disease: Long-term complications. *Nat. Cancer Institute Monogr.* 1973; 36:447–454.

DeVita, V., Serpick, A., Carbone, P.: Combination chemotherapy and the treatment of advanced Hodgkin's disease. *Annals Intern. Med.* 73:881–895, 1970.

Dolan, D.M., Coltman, C.A., Jr., Moon, T.E.: Second malignancies complicating Hodgkin's disease: The southwest oncology group experience. *Cancer Clinical Trials* 1:27, 1978.

Dresser, R.K., Golomb, H.M., Ultmann, J.E., et al.: Prognostic classification of Hodgkin's disease in pathologic Stage III, based on anatomic consideration. *Blood* 49(6):883–893, 1977.

Duncan, P.R., Checa, F., Gowing, N.F., et al.: Extranodal non-Hodgkin's lymphoma present in the testicle: A clinical and pathologic study of 24 cases. *Cancer* 45(7):1578–1584, 1980.

Edelstyn, G.A., Robertson, J.H., Newsholme, G.A., et al.: British national lymphoma investigation: Initial treatment of Stage III Hodgkin's disease. Comparison of radiotherapy with combined chemotherapy. *Lancet* 2:991–995, 1976.

Farber, L.R., Prosnitz, L.R., Cadman, E.C., et al.: Curative potential of combined modality therapy for advanced Hodgkin's disease. *Cancer* 46:1509–1517, 1980.

Foucar, K., McKenna, R.N., Bloomfield, C.D., et al.: Therapy-related leukemia: A panmyelosis. *Cancer* 43:1285–1296, 1979.

Frazer, R.W., Chism, S.E., Stern, R., et al.: Clinical course of early extranodal non-Hodgkin's lymphomas. *Int. J. Radiation Oncol. Biol. Phys.* 5(2):177–183, 1979.

Frei, E., Luce, J.K., Gamble, J.F., et al.: Combination chemotherapy in advanced Hodgkin's disease: Induction and maintenance of remission. *Annals Intern. Med.* 79:376–382, 1973.

Fuller, L.M., Gamble, J.F., Villouscuaze, W.S., et al.: Evaluation of the significance of prognostic factors in Stage III Hodgkin's disease treated with MOPP and radiotherapy. *Cancer* 45:1352–1363, 1980.

Fuller, L.M., Madoc-Jones, H., Gamble, J.F., et al.: New assessment of the prognostic significance of histopathology in Hodgkin's disease for laparotomy-negative Stage I and Stage II patients. *Cancer* 39(5):2174–2182, 1977.

Fuller, L.M., Madoc-Jones, H., Hagemeister, F.B., et al.: Further follow-up of results of treatment in 90 laparotomy-negative Stage I and II Hodgkin's disease patients: Significance of mediastinal and nonmediastinal presentations. *Int. J. Radiation Oncol. Biol. Phys.* 6:799–808, 1980.

Glatstein, E.: Radiotherapy in Hodgkin's disease: past achievements and future progress. *Cancer* 39:837–843, 1977.

Glatstein, E., Donaldson, S.S., Rosenberg, S.E., et al.: Combined modality therapy in malignant lymphomas. *Cancer Treatment Rep.* 61:1199–1207, 1977.

Glatstein, E., Fuks, Z., Goffinet, D.R., et al.: Non-Hodgkin's lymphomas of Stage III extent: Is total lymphoid irradiation appropriate treatment? *Cancer* 37:2806–2812, 1976.

Glatstein, E., McHardy-Young, S., Brast, N., et al.: Alterations in serum Thyrotropin (TSH) and thyroid function following radiotherapy in patients with malignant lymphoma. *J. Clin. Endocrinol. Metab.* 32:833–841, 1971.

Goffinet, D.R., Warnicki, R., Donnick, N.E., et al.: Clinical and surgical (laparotomy) evaluation of patients with non-Hodgkin's lymphomas. *Cancer Treatment Rep.* 61:981–992, 1977.

Golomb, H.M., Sweet, D.L., Ultmann, J.E., et al.: Importance of substaging of Stage III Hodgkin's disease. *Semin. Oncol.* 7:136–143, 1980.

Goodman, R., Mauch, P., Piro, A., et al.: Stages II-B and III-B Hodgkin's disease: Results of combined modality treatment. *Cancer* 40(1):84–89, July 1977.

Goodman, R.L., Piro, A.J., Hellman, S.: Can pelvic irradiation be omitted in patients with pathologic Stages I-A and II-A Hodgkin's disease? *Cancer* 37:2834–2839, 1976.

Harrison, D.T., et al.: Combined modality therapy for advanced diffuse lymphocytic and histiocytic lymphomas. *Cancer* 42(4):1697–1704, 1978.

Hellman, S.: An evaluation of total nodal irradiation as treatment for Stage III-A Hodgkin's disease. *Cancer* 43(4):1255–1261, 1979.

Hellman, S., Mauch, P., Goodman, R.L., et al.: The place of radiation therapy in the treatment of Hodgkin's disease. *Cancer* 42:971, 1978.

Hoppe, R.T., Coleman, C.N., Kaplan, H.S., et al.: Hodgkin's disease, pathologic Stage I–II: The prognostic importance of initial sites of disease and extent of mediastinal involvement. *Proceedings Am. Soc. Clin. Oncol.* 21:471, 1980.

Hoppe, R.T., Cox, R.S., Rosenberg, S.A.: Prognostic factors in pathologic Stage III-A Hodgkin's disease (abstracts). *Proceedings Am. Soc. Clin. Oncol.* 20:429, 1979.

Hoppe, R.T., Portlock, C.S., Glatstein, E., et al.: Alternating chemotherapy and irradiation in the treatment of advanced Hodgkin's disease. *Cancer* 43(2):472–481, 1979.

Hoppe, R.T., Rosenberg, S.A., Kaplan, H.S., et al.: Prognostic factors in pathological Stage IIIa Hodgkin's disease. *Cancer* 46:1240–1246, 1980.

Johnson, R.E., Canellos, G.P., Young, R.C., et al.: Chemotherapy (cyclosphosphamide, vincristine, and prednisone) versus radiotherapy (TBI) in Stage III-IV poorly differentiated lymphocytic lymphoma. *Cancer Treatment Rep.* 62:321–325, 1978.

Johnson, R.E., Thomas, L.B., Schneiderman, M., et al.: Preliminary experience with total nodal irradiation in Hodgkin's disease. *Radiology* 96:603, 1970.

Johnson, R.E., Zimbler, H., Berard, C.W., et al.: Radiotherapy results for nodular sclerosing Hodgkin's disease after clinical staging. *Cancer* 39:1439–1444, 1977.

Jones, A.: Transient radiation myelopathy with reference to Lhermitte's sign of electrical parathesia. *Br. J. Radiol.* 37:727–744, 1964.

Jones, S.E., Fuks, Z., Kaplan, H.S.: Non-Hodgkin's lymphomas. V, results of radiotherapy. *Cancer* 32:682–691, 1973.

Kaplan, H.S.: Evidence for a tumoricidal dose level in the radiotherapy of Hodgkin's disease. *Cancer Res.* 26:1221–1224, 1966.

Kaplan, H.S.: *The Harvey Lectures.* Series 64, 1968–1969, New York, Academic Press, 1970:215–259.

Kaplan, H.S.: *Hodgkin's Disease,* 2nd edition. Cambridge, Massachusetts, Harvard University Press, 1980.

Kaplan, H.S., Rosenberg, S.A.: Current status of clinical trials: Stanford experience, 1962–72. *National Cancer Institute Monographs* 36:363–371, 1973.

Karzmark, C.J.: Physical and dosimetric aspects of the radiotherapy of malignant lymphomas: II. The inverted-Y technique. *Radiology* 96:619–629, 1970.

Kelly, M.G., O'Gara, R.W., Gadekar, K., et al.: Carcinogenic activity of a new antitumor agent, N-Isopropyl-a-(2-methylhydrazino)-p-toluamide, Hydrochloride (NSC-77213). *Cancer Chemotherapy Rep.* 39:77–80, 1964.

Krikorian, J.G., Portlock, C.S., Rosenberg, S.A., et al.: Hodgkin's disease, Stages I and II, occurring below the diaphragm. *Cancer* 43:1866–1871, 1979.

Kun, L.E., DeVita, V.T., Jr., Young, R.C., et al.: Treatment of Hodgkin's disease using intensive chemotherapy followed by irradiation. *Int. J. Radiation Oncol. Biol. Phys.* 1:619–626, 1976.

Landberg, T., Liden, K., Forslo, H.: Split-course radiation therapy of mediastinal Hodgkin's disease: TSD and CRE concepts. *Acta Radiol. Ther. Phys. Biol.* 12:33, 1973.

LeFoch, O., Donaldson, S.S., Kaplan, H.S.: Pregnancy following cophoropexy and total nodal irradiation in women with Hodgkin's disease. *Cancer* 38:2263–2268, 1976.

Levi, J.A., Wiernik, P.H.: Limited extranodal Hodgkin's disease: Unfavorable prognosis and therapeutic implications. *Am. J. Med.* 63:365–372, 1977.

Levi, J.A., Wiernik, P.H.: The therapeutic implications of splenic involvement in Stage III-A Hodgkin's disease. *Cancer* 39(5):2158–2165, 1977.

Levitt, S.H., Bloomfield, C.D., Lee, C.K., et al.: Extended field radiotherapy in non-Hodgkin's lymphoma. *Radiology* 118(2):457–459, 1976.

Lutz, W.R., Larsen, R.D.: Technique to match mantle and paraaortic fields. *Int. J. Radiation Oncol. Biol. Phys.* 5(2):159, 1979.

Mauch, P., Goodman, R., Hellman, S.: The significance of mediastinal involvement in early stage Hodgkin's disease. *Cancer* 42:1039–1045, 1978.

Mauch, P., Goodman, R., Rosenthal, D.S., et al.: An evaluation of total nodal irradiation as treatment for Stage IIIa Hodgkin's disease. *Cancer* 43:1255–1261, 1979.

Mauch, P., Hellman, S.: Supradiaphragmatic Hodgkin's disease: Is there a role for MOPP chemotherapy in patients with bulky mediastinal disease? *Int. J. Radiation Oncol. Biol. Phys.* 6:947–949, 1980.

Miller, T.P., Jones, S.E.: Is there a role for radiotherapy in localized diffuse lymphomas? *Cancer Chemotherapy Pharmacol.* 4(2):67–70, 1980.

Murphy, S.B.: Management of childhood non-Hodgkin's lymphoma. *Cancer Treatment Rep.* 61:1161–1173, 1977.

Page, V., Gardner, A., Karzmark, C.J.: Physical and dosimetric aspects of the radiotherapy of malignant lymphomas: I. The mantle technique. *Radiology* 96:609–618, 1970.

Paladugu, R.R., Bearman, R.M., Rappaport, H.: Malignant lymphoma with primary manifestation in the gonad: A clinicopathological study of 38 patients. *Cancer* 45:561–571, 1980.

Patchefsky, A.R., Brodovsky, H., Southard, M., et al.: Hodgkin's disease: A clinical and pathologic study of 235 cases. *Cancer* 32:150–161, 1973.

Piro, A.J., Wiess, D.R., Hellman, S.: Mediastinal Hodgkin's disease: A possible danger for intubation anesthesia. *Int. J. Radiation Oncol. Biol. Phys.* 1:415–419, 1976.

Portlock, C.S., Rosenberg, S.A., Glatstein, E.: Impact of salvage treatment on initial relapses in patients with Hodgkin's disease, Stages I-III. *Blood* 51:825–833, 1978.

Portlock, C.S., Rosenberg, S.A., Glatstein, E., et al.: Treatment of advanced non-Hodgkin's lymphomas with favorable histologies: Preliminary results of a prospective trial. *Blood* 45(5):747–756, 1976.

Proceedings of the Symposium on Contemporary Issues in Hodgkin's Disease, Biology, Staging and Treatment. *Cancer Treatment Report* 66:601–1071, 1982.

Prosnitz, L.R., Farber, L.R., Fisher, J.J., et al.: Long-term remission with combined modality therapy for advanced Hodgkin's disease. *Cancer* 37(6):2826–2833, 1976.

Prosnitz, L.R., Montalvo, R.L., Fischer, D.B., et al.: Treatment of Stage III-A Hodgkin's disease: Is radiotherapy alone adequate? *Int. J. Radiation Oncol. Biol. Phys.* 4:781–787, 1978.

Rappaport, H., Winter, W.J., Hicks, E.B.: Follicular lymphoma: A reevaluation of its position in the scheme of malignant lymphomas, based on a survey of 253 cases. *Cancer* 9:792–821, 1956.

Rodgers, R.W., Fuller, L.M., Hagemeister, F.B., et al.: Reassessment of diagnostic factors in Stage III-A and III-B Hodgkin's disease treated with MOPP and radiotherapy. *Cancer* 47:2196–2203, 1981.

Rodichok, L.D., Harper, G.R., Ruckdeschel, J.C., et al.: Early diagnosis of spinal epidural metastases. *Am. J. Med.* 70(6):1181–1188, 1981.

Rosenberg, S.A.: Management of Hodgkin's disease. *Northeast J. Med.* 299:1246–1247, 1978.

Rosenberg, S.A., Kaplan, H.S., Glatstein, E.G., et al.: Combined modality therapy of Hodgkin's disease: A report on the Stanford trials. *Cancer* 42:991–1000, 1978.

Schein, P.S., Chabner, B.A., Canellos, J.P., et al.: Potential for prolonged disease-free survival following combination chemotherapy of non-Hodgkin's disease. *Blood* 43:181–189, 1974.

Sieber, S.M., Correa, P., Delgard, D.W., et al.: Carcinogenic and other adverse effects of Procarbazine in nonhumans. *Cancer Res.* 38:2125–2134, 1978.

Sherins, R.J., DeVita, V.T.: Effect of drug treatment for lymphoma on male reproduction capacity: Studies of men in remission after therapy. *Annals Intern. Med.* 79:216–220, 1973.

Slanina, J., Musskoff, K., Rahner, T., et al.: Long-term side effects in irradiated patients with Hodgkin's disease. *Int. J. Radiology Biol. Phys.* 2:1–19, 1977.

Speiser, B., Rubin, P., Casarett, G.: Aspermia following lower trunkal irradiation in Hodgkin's disease. *Cancer* 32:692–698, 1973.

Stein, R.S., Golomb, H.M., Ultmann, J.E., et al.: Anatomic substages of Stage III Hodgkin's disease: A collaborative study. *Proceedings Am. Soc. Clin. Oncol.* 20:438, 1979.

Stein, R.S., Golomb, H.M., Wiernik, P.H., et al.: Anatomic substages of Stage III-A Hodgkin's disease: Follow-up of a collaborative study. *Cancer Treatment Rep.* 66(4):733–741, 1982.

Stein, R.S., Hilborn, R.M., Flexner, J.M., et al.: Anatomical substages of Stage III Hodgkin's disease: Implications for staging, therapy and experimental design. *Cancer* 42(2):429–436, 1978.

Stewart, J.R., Cohn, K.E., Fajardo, L.F., et al.: Radiation-induced heart disease: A study of 25 patients. *Radiology* 89:302–310, 1967.

Strauss, D.J., Myers, J., Passe, S., et al.: The eight-drug/radiation therapy program (MOPP/ABVD/RT) for advanced Hodgkin's disease: A follow-up report. *Cancer* 46:233–240, 1980.

Sweet, D.L., Golomb, H.M.: The treatment of histiocytic lymphoma. *Semin. Oncol.* 7:302–309, 1980.

Thar, T.L., Million, R.R., Hausner, R.J., et al.: Hodgkin's disease, Stages I & II: Relationship of recurrence to size of disease, radiation dose, and number of sites involved. *Cancer* 43:1101–1105, 1979.

Thar, T.L., Million, R.R., Noyes, W.D.: Total body irradiation in non-Hodgkin's lymphoma. *Int. J. Radiation Oncol. Biol. Phys.* 5(2):171–176, 1979.

Toland, D.M., Coltman, C.A., Jr., Moon, T.E.: Second malignancies complicating Hodgkin's disease: The southwest oncology group experience. *Cancer Clinical Trials* 1:27, 1978.

Toonkel, L.M., Fuller, L.M., Gamble, J.F. et al.: Laparotomy staged I and II non-Hodgkin's lymphomas: Preliminary results of radiotherapy and adjunctive chemotherapy. *Cancer* 45:249–260, 1980.

Torte, F.M., Dorfman, R.F., Rosenberg, S.A., et al.: The changing significance of histology in Hodgkin's disease. *Proceedings Am. Cancer Res., Am. Soc. Clin. Oncol.* 19–20:401, 1979.

Valentjas, E., Baratte, A., Macelwen, T.J.: Mediastinal involvement in early Stage Hodgkin's disease: Response to treatment and pattern of relapse. *Eur. J. Cancer* 126:1065–1068, 1976.

Weller, S.A., Glatstein, E., Castallino, R.A., et al.: Initial relapse in previously treated Hodgkin's disease-II: Retrograde transdiaphragmatic extension. *Int. J. Radiation Oncol. Biol. Phys.* 2:863–872, 1977.

Young, R.C., Johnson, R.E., Canellos, R.P., et al.: Advanced lymphocytic lymphoma: Randomized comparisons of chemotherapy and radiotherapy, alone or in combination. *Cancer Treatment Rep.* 61:1153–1159, 1977.

8

Childhood Lymphomas

Raymond Tannous, M.D.

Introduction

Childhood lymphomas, like adult lymphomas, are classically divided into two major subgroups: non-Hodgkin's lymphomas (NHL) and Hodgkin's disease. While childhood Hodgkin's disease does not differ from that seen in early adulthood, childhood NHLs are dramatically different from common adult NHLs by pathological type, epidemiology, natural history, and prognosis.

Non-Hodgkin's Lymphoma

This heading covers a heterogeneous group of lymphomatous and histiocytic malignancies. The imprecision of the heading reflects the long-standing difficulties in classifying and treating these relatively rare diseases in both children and adults.

Epidemiology and Incidence

NHL occurs in 7.5 per 1 million children annually and affects mostly males. With some exceptions, NHLs are sporadic and their etiology is unknown. Exceptions include the higher incidence of NHL in patients with immunodeficiency (Wiskott-Aldrich syndrome, X-linked agammaglobulinemia, severe combined immunodeficiency, common variable immunodeficiency, and ataxia telangiectasia), patients with X-linked lymphoproliferative syndrome, survivors of other primary cancers previously treated with alkylating agents, and recipients of organ transplants. NHLs are endemic in Africa and underprivileged Middle Eastern countries where viral infections such as Ebstein-Barr virus and parasitic infections such as malaria and intestinal parasites prevail.

Cytogenetic studies have demonstrated that patients with Burkitt's lymphomas have an extra band at the end of the long arm of chromosome 14 (14 q^+), often resulting from a balanced translocation of genetic material from the long arm of chromosome 8 (8 q^-).

Pathological Classification and Staging

Appropriate classification and staging of a malignancy require standard and reproducible clinical and pathological criteria which have therapeutic and/or prognostic implications. Unfortunately, differing classifications, small patient populations, and heterogeneity in treatment and staging by various treatment centers prevent comparisons and hamper progress in our understanding of NHL.

NHL can be classified morphologically (Rappaport), by cell type and degree of differentiation (cell surface markers), or by using both morphological cell type and characteristics (Lukes and Collins). No morphological classification satisfies fully the criteria cited above, and the prognostic and therapeutic implications of cell type and differentiation await further definition. Details of prevailing classifications can be found in the pathological discussion in this book. We will simply outline the various NHLs seen in children by both cell type (as defined by cell surface markers) and by their most commonly used descriptive terminology.

Only 1–2% of childhood NHLs are low-grade follicular (nodular) lymphomas. The remaining NHLs are high-grade diffuse, and comprise three major groups. T-cell NHL (lymphoblastic, convoluted lymphocytic) is seen in 40% of cases. B-cell NHLs (small noncleaved) are seen in another 40% of cases and include endemic Burkitt's, nonendemic Burkitt's, and non-Burkitt's lymphomas. The third group, usually called histiocytic or large cell, is heterogeneous in cell origin, being mostly B cell but also occasionally T cell, non-B non-T cell, or even true histiocytic. The latter group is seen in 7–23% of cases.

Staging schemas are numerous and their lack of homogeneity will most likely remain until prognostic factors are further defined. Factors that may contribute to poor prognosis are related to cell morphology, cell type, site of primary, resectability, degree of dissemination, central nervous system involvement, and bone marrow involvement. Among the three commonly used staging systems shown in Table 1, the system

Table 1
Staging of Childhood NHL

CCSG	St. Jude Children's Hospital	Sloan-Kettering Cancer Center
Good prognosis (localized)	I Single lesion (excluding abdominal, mediastinal, epidural, and paraspinal primaries)	Single lesion
	II Single lesion + regional adenopathy Gastrointestinal lesion ± mesenteric node involvement (resectable)	Single lesion + regional adenopathy
Poor prognosis nonlymphoblastic lymphoblastic	Two extranodal lesions ± adenopathy on one side of diaphragm Two or more nodal lesions on one side of diaphragm	
	III Stage II with disease on both sides of diaphragm Any intrathoracic lesion Extensive (nonresectable) abdominal disease Paraspinal or epidural sites	Two or more lesions on both sides of diaphragm Extensive intrathoracic disease Extensive abdominal disease
	IV Bone marrow (≤25%) and/or central nervous system (CNS) involvement	Bone marrow (≤25%) and/or central nervous system (CNS) involvement
Leukemia-lymphoma syndrome	Bone marrow (>25%)	Bone marrow (>25%)

used by the Childrens Cancer Study Group (CCSG) accounts best for the prognostic factors and thus divides NHL patients into four groups:

(1) Good prognosis localized (Stage I and most Stage II by the St. Jude Children's Research Hospital and the Memorial Sloan-Kettering Cancer Center schemas)
- Gastrointestinal primary with or without regional node involvement. Completely resected.
- Waldeyer's ring with or without cervical and/or supraclavicular lymph node involvement.
- Any single extralymphatic site with or without regional node involvement. Bone and mediastinal primaries excluded.
- Nodal disease limited to a single or two adjacent lymphatic regions.

(2) Poor prognosis nonlymphoblastic, (Stage III, most Stage IV, and some Stage II by the St. Jude and Sloan-Kettering schemas)
- Any localized nonlymphoblastic NHL involving mediastinum or cortical bone.
- Nonlocalized nonlymphoblastic NHL.

(3) Poor prognosis lymphoblastic (Stages III and IV by St. Jude staging)
- Mediastinal primary lymphoblastic.
- Nonlocalized lymphoblastic.

(4) Leukemia-lymphoma syndrome
- Patients with >25% marrow involvement and mediastinal mass or massive adenopathy or organomegaly, and initial WBC > 50,000 or hemoglobin ≥ 10 gm/dl.

Presenting Clinical Symptoms

Older male predominance is seen in most childhood NHL. Unexplained fever occurs in one-third. Other presenting symptoms vary with the primary site and the type of NHL in question. Lymphoblastic lymphomas are likely to present with an anterior mediastinal mass and/or anterior cervical adenopathy, supraclavicular adenopathy, or pleural effusion. Possible symptoms include dyspnea, superior vena cava syndrome, wheezing, and coughing. Symptoms of increased intracranial pressure may be due to venous obstruction and/or central nervous system (CNS) involvement.

Endemic or African Burkitt's lymphoma has distinct clinical features, often manifesting itself with a rapidly growing jaw or orbital mass. When intraabdominal, it may arise from kidneys, ovaries, or retroperitoneal structures. Only rarely does endemic Burkitt's lymphoma involve bone, testes, breast, thyroid, parotid, or skin. Lymph node and bone marrow involvement is very rare, but CNS involvement is a frequent complication during relapses.

Nonendemic Burkitt's lymphoma differs from the endemic form by its prevalence in the abdomen where it involves most commonly the Peyer's patches of the ileocecal region or the mesenteric lymph nodes. Common presenting clinical features include abdominal pain, vomiting, and the presence of an abdominal mass. It is the most common cause of intussusception in children older than 6 years. Cervical lymph nodes are another common primary site. Both bone marrow and CNS involvement are common in nonendemic NHLs, with the exception of those localized to the gastrointestinal tract and which are totally resected.

The small noncleaved (non-Burkitt's) NHLs present most often in the lymph nodes. The frequency with which bone marrow, CNS, skeletal system, liver, spleen, skin, and lungs are involved is similar to that found in nonendemic Burkitt's.

The large cell lymphomas are more often extranodal in origin and may occur in the nasopharynx, tonsil, lung, mediastinum, bone, gonad, skin, and other soft tissues. They very rarely occur in the gastrointestinal tract. Bone marrow and CNS involvement may also occur.

Nodular lymphomas are rare and are usually localized to lymph nodes. Bone marrow and CNS involvement are rare. Prognosis is good unless transformation into a diffuse large cell type occurs.

Evaluation

NHLs are usually rapidly progressive. They have high proliferative activity and disseminate quickly. Consequently, early detection of metabolic anomalies (hyperuricemia, hyperphosphatemia, hypocalcemia, lactic acidosis) and impaired renal and liver functions is necessary in patients with NHL. Patients with large tumors, particularly those with Burkitt's lymphoma, are likely to develop these abnormalities before and more surely after therapy is instituted (the so-called "tumor lysis" syndrome). Serum lactic dehydrogenase and copper may also serve as nonspecific markers of tumor load and activity.

Diagnostic and staging procedures must be performed rapidly, and therapy preferably instituted within 72 hours. Studies should include serum blood urea nitrogen, creatinine, uric acid, electrolytes including phosphorus, calcium, and potassium, lactic dehydrogenase, serum copper, hemoglobin, white blood count, and differential. Bone marrow aspiration from at least two sites is necessary to assess the presence and percentage of lymphoma cells. When involved by the malignant process, bone marrow samples are ideal to study cell morphology, cytogenetic anomalies, biochemical cell markers such as PAS, nonspecific esterase, myeloperoxidase, and terminal deoxytransferase stains) as well as to define cell type through use of cell markers (rosetting with sheep erythrocytes, presence of immunoglobulins, and specific surface antigens). Cerebral spinal fluid examination including cell count, differential, and morphology on preparations obtained by cytospin or millipore filter techniques is required to detect the presence of CNS involvement.

Radiological studies should include chest roentgenograms, bone survey, and scans of the liver and spleen. Special indications include head and abdominal computerized axial tomography, gastrointestinal contrast studies, an intravenous pyelogram, bilateral lower extremity lymphangiography, and whole body ^{67}Ga citrate scan.

A diagnostic biopsy specimen should be obtained from the most accessible location in disseminated cases or following complete resection in localized ones. Abdominal gastrointestinal primaries should be resected *en bloc* with the distal ileum, cecum, appendix, and associated mesentery included in the resection whenever the tumor is resectable. In larger tumors, tumor reduction may decrease the possibility of the metabolic complications mentioned earlier. Visual and palpatory exploration of the abdominal organs, retroperitoneal structures along with removal of palpable lymph nodes, and liver biopsy will provide better staging. Touch preparations and frozen unfixed tumor tissues are necessary for cytochemical stains, cell markers, and occasionally electron microscopic studies. It should be emphasized that patients with poor prognosis and those with widespread disease often require immediate therapy and should not undergo extensive staging procedures.

Therapy

Two major therapeutic aspects must be considered simultaneously by the physician. These relate to tumor control and to complications of tumor growth and therapy.

Surgery

Besides its diagnostic value, surgery is of benefit in localized NHL. The effect of surgery on survival is best illustrated in abdominal Burkitt's lymphoma where completely and almost completely resected tumors fared significantly better than unresectable ones. Wherever possible, total or at least 90% resection should be attempted. In disseminated tumors, surgery has no proven role, and while debulking may decrease the likelihood of metabolic complications, this should not be undertaken if it increases the surgical risk.

Chemotherapy

The use of multiagent chemotherapy has produced the most dramatic improvement in disease-free survival. Several effective combinations have been described. Unfortunately, few randomized studies were undertaken to select the most effective and least toxic therapies. Commonly used combinations include the COMP regimen of Ziegler (combination of cyclophosphamide, Oncovin, methotrexate, and prednisone), the LSA_2-L_2 regimen of Wollner (a more intensive combination of ten agents), the equally intensive Berlin-Frankfurt-Muenster acute lymphoblastic leukemia protocol (BFM), and several modifications of each.

All these regimens are effective in good-prognosis NHL, achieving 80–100% disease-free survival (DFS). Since survival was similar with COMP-like and LSA_2-L_2-like regimens in the randomized CCSG study 551, the Children's Cancer Study Group has opted for the less toxic COMP-like regimen. These patients are currently randomized to receive either 6 months or 18 months of maintenance therapy, and preliminary data suggests no difference in outcome.

In nonlocalized and poor-prognosis NHL, the LSA_2-L_2 regimen was a major breakthrough. More recently similar results were achieved with COMP-like and BFM regimens. LSA_2-L_2 therapy was found effective in all types of NHL by some (Wollner, Miser, Sullivan) with a 70% overall DFS. Less favorable results may be seen in patients with cortical bone primaries and in those with extensive bone marrow involvement. The LSA_2-L_2 versus COMP randomized CCSG study 551 yielded similar survival rates with both regimens; however, patients with lymphoblastic (presumably T-cell) histology fared better with LSA_2-L_2 therapy (80% 2–year DFS when compared to 25% DFS with COMP). The nonlymphoblastic NHL patients, on the other hand, fared better with COMP-like therapy (60% DFS) than with LSA_2-L_2 (30% DFS). These results are in agreement with those reported by others (Vecchi, Pichler). Preliminary data suggests that BFM therapy may be more effective for null and T-cell NHL as opposed to B-cell disease.

Radiotherapy

NHLs are responsive to radiation therapy; however, the role of radiation therapy in improving survival remains unknown. In localized totally resectable intraabdominal disease, up to 60% relapses were reported after radiotherapy. Conversely, 80–100% DFS is seen with COMP-like and LSA_2-L_2 chemotherapy with or without radiotherapy. In patients with unresectable disease, because of location or extent, radiotherapy is often recommended though its role also remains undefined. Thus radiotherapy must be considered with caution since it may prevent or delay chemotherapy and because of its acute and long-term toxicities.

In summary, indications for radiotherapy in either localized or disseminated NHL are not based on solid survival data from randomized trials. Such therapy should perhaps be limited to patients with residual disease following induction chemotherapy and to patients with life-threatening complications such as upper airway obstruction, or to prevent CNS complications in patients with hyperleukocytosis (WBC $> 100{,}000/mm^3$). Radiotherapy is also indicated in patients with CNS involvement. Its effectiveness in CNS prophylaxis has also been demonstrated, although such prophylaxis may be attainable in most patients with intrathecal chemotherapy alone.

CNS Prophylaxis

Prophylaxis of CNS involvement is necessary in all patients with NHL except in those with localized gastrointestinal disease. While a combination of cranial radiation and intrathecal methotrexate is effective, administration of intrathecal methotrexate during induction and maintenance therapy without cranial radiation has resulted in only 6% isolated CNS relapses. The improved results in leukemic CNS prophylaxis using the Bleyer intrathecal methotrexate regimen may further improve results in NHL CNS prophylaxis.

Metabolic Emergencies

As mentioned earlier, metabolic complications including hyperuricemia, hyperkalemia, and hyperphosphatemia with hypocalcemia may occur individually or in combination (acute tumor lysis syndrome). Hyperuricemia is, for example, the most common cause of renal failure in these patients. Metabolic abnormalities are more likely to be seen in patients with a large tumor burden and most often in Burkitt's NHL and T-cell lymphoma/leukemia syndrome. The best therapy for the tumor lysis syndrome is prevention, using hydration, alkalinization of the urine, and allopurinol administration to decrease uric acid production and prevent renal failure. Urine output should be maintained at 100 ml/m^2/hr and urine pH at 7.0 to 7.5. Dialysis should be considered in patients with renal failure or K+ $\geq$ 6 mEq/dl, phosphorus $\geq$ 10 mg/dl, symptomatic hypocalcemia, or fluid overload despite diuretic therapy.

Other metabolic abnormalities include hyponatremia resulting from salt depletion (due to diarrhea, vomiting, or excessive diuresis), inappropriate antidiuretic hormone production, adrenal insufficiency, hypercalcemia, or other large osmotic loads that prevent renal tubular reabsorption. Hypokalemia (because of excessive gastrointestinal or renal losses), hypercalcemia, and lactic acidosis have also been described. These metabolic abnormalities should be treated appropriately, such as by replacement of depleted electrolytes or restrictive fluid therapy for inappropriate antidiuretic hormone secretion.

Summary

Childhood NHLs are characterized by rapid progression and early dissemination to various sites including some sanctuaries such as the central nervous system where systemic therapy is not efficacious.

Rapid progression dictates an expeditious initial evaluation to establish the diagnosis and any metabolic abnormalities. However, a precise diagnosis is necessary, including adequate pathological classification and staging, if the patient is to receive a custom-tailored rather than a standard across-the-board therapy.

Early dissemination dictates that multiagent chemotherapy be given to every NHL patient irrespective of class or stage, and central nervous system prophylaxis be given to all but those with completely resectable localized gastrointestinal disease. More randomized studies are needed to define the most effective and least toxic therapies for different stages and classes of NHL. Such studies require large numbers of patients and consequently should include several centers. In the absence of an ongoing study, we would presently recommend 6 months of the less toxic COMP therapy for all good-prognosis patients, a full course of COMP for nonlymphoblastic poor-prognosis patients, and either LSA_2-L_2 or BFM regimens for those with poor-prognosis lymphoblastic NHL. Surgical removal is recommended whenever possible. Efficacy of radiotherapy to primary site and bulky disease should be further investigated.

Once initiated, most of the therapy can be provided by the family physician, as we have demonstrated at The University of Iowa. However, initial evaluation, staging, and classification can most efficiently and rapidly be performed in a cancer center.

Selected Reading

Bleyer, W.A.: Clinical pharmacology of intrathecal methotrexate. II. An improved dosage regimen derived from age-related pharmacokinetics. *Cancer Treatment Rep.* 61:1419, 1977.

Coccia, P.F., Kersey, J.H., Gajl-Peczalska, K.J., et al.: Prognostic significance of surface marker analysis in childhood non-Hodgkin's lymphoproliferative malignancies. *Am. J. Hematol.* 1:405–417, 1976.

Cohen, L.F., Balow, J.E., Magrath, I.T., et al.: Acute tumor lysis syndrome. A review of 37 patients with Burkitt's lymphoma. *Am. J. Med.* 68:486, 1980.

Jenkin, R.D.T., Anderson, J.R., Chilcote, R.: Pediatric non-Hodgkin's lymphomas: The Children's Cancer Study Group experience—an interim report, in Rosenberg, S.A., Kaplan, H.S. (eds.): *Malignant Lymphomas: Etiology, Immunology, Pathology, Treatment.* New York, Academic Press, 1982.

Jereb, B., Wollner, N., Kosloff, C., et al.: The role of local radiation in the treatment of non-Hodgkin lymphoma in children. *Med. Pediatr. Oncol.* 9:157, 1981.

Levine, P.H., Kamaraju, L.S., Connelly, R.R., et al.: The American Burkitt's lymphoma registry: Eight years experience. *Cancer* 49:1016, 1982.

Lukes, R.J., Collins, R.D.: Immunologic characterization of human malignant lymphomas. *Cancer* 34:1488, 1974.

Murphy, S.B.: Classification, staging, and end results of treatment of childhood non-Hodgkin's lymphomas: Dissimilarities from lymphomas in adults. *Semin. Oncol.* 7:332, 1980.

Nelson, D.F., Cassady, J.R., Traggis, D., et al.: The role of radiation therapy in localized resectable intestinal non-Hodgkin's lymphoma in children. *Cancer* 38:89, 1977.

Perry, M.C., Hoagland, H.C., Wagoner, R.D.: Uric acid nephropathy. *J.A.M.A.* 236:961, 1976.

Pichler, E., Jürgenssen O.-A., Radaszkiewicz, T., et al.: Results of LSA_2-L_2 therapy in 26 children with non-Hodgkin's lymphoma. *Cancer* 50:2740–2746, 1982.

Quinn, J.J., Taylor, C.R., Swanson, V., et al.: Childhood leukemia and lymphoma: Correlation of clinical features with immunological and morphological studies. *Med. Pediatr. Oncol.* 7:35, 1979.

Rappaport, H., Winter, W., Hicks, E.: Follicular lymphoma. *Cancer* 9:792, 1956.

St. Muller-Weihrich, Henze, G., Kornhuber, B., et al.: The BFM study 1976/80 on childhood non-Hodgkin's lymphoma (NHL): Prognostic relevance of clinical stage and histology/immunology. *Proceedings of the International Conference on Malignant Lymphomas,* abstract, p. 19, 1981.

Vecchi, V., Pession, A., Serra, L., et al.: Non-Hodgkin's lymphoma in children: Results of treatment with the modified LSA_2-L_2 protocol. *Med. Pediatr. Oncol.* 9:483, 1981.
Wollner, N.: LSA_2-L_2 in childhood non-Hodgkin's lymphoma, in Rosenberg, S.A., Kaplan, H.S. (eds.): *Malignant Lymphomas: Etiology, Immunology, Pathology, Treatment*. New York, Academic Press, 1982.
Zea, J.M., Exelby, P.R., Wollner, N.: Abdominal non-Hodgkin's lymphoma in childhood. *J. Pediatr. Surg.* 11:363, 1976.
Ziegler, J.L.: Burkitt's lymphoma. *N. Engl. J. Med.* 305:735, 1981.

9

Natural History of the Lymphomas

Matthew N. Stein, M.D., Michael P. Corder, M.D.

Introduction

The natural history of the lymphomas of necessity involves the description of the course of treated as well as untreated disease. Since lymphomatous diseases were first treated with orthovoltage radiation early in this century, their course has gradually been changing. A complete description of their natural history is interwoven with the changes in outcome that have occurred as a result of therapy.

Attention will be given to historical perspective, clinical presentation of disease, and alteration of disease course in Hodgkin's lymphoma and the major subgroups of the non-Hodgkin's lymphomas. The Rappaport system of histopathology for non-Hodgkin's lymphoma will be utilized with parenthetic expression of the newer National Cancer Institute Working Formulation of non-Hodgkin's Lymphoma for Clinical Usage (Working Formulation).

Histopathological diagnosis is critical to the understanding and prediction of disease outcome in both Hodgkin's and non-Hodgkin's lymphoma. Even in the hands of the most experienced hematopathologists, this is a difficult task. Under ideal circumstances, with concurrent review and open discussion of diagnostic possibilities, reproducibility of diagnostic results will approach 90%. In less experienced hands without open review this concordance rate, when compared with the lymphoma panel of the National Cancer Institute, is much less. Therefore, it is critical that the discussion of natural history, treatment, and predictability of outcome be understood in that light and conclusions drawn appropriate to these limitations.

Hodgkin's Lymphomas

The historical prelude to the assessment and treatment of Hodgkin's lymphoma begins with the original description by Thomas Hodgkin in 1832 of pathological lymphadenopathy and splenomegaly associated with lymphomatous disease. Throughout the 19th century, accumulated pathological descriptions of lymphatic malignancy added credence to the uniqueness of Hodgkin's observations. As will be indicated in the discussion of the non-Hodgkin's lymphomas, pathological separation of the two entities began in the 1920s with the description of the non-Hodgkin's lymphoma as a separate group.

Pathological classifications have undergone transition and solidification with the current system from the Rye Conference in the late 1960s. Though problems with histopathological concordance do exist, in the hands of experienced hematopathologists they are less than those of the non-Hodgkin's lymphomas.

The natural history of the Hodgkin's lymphomas and the changes that have occurred over the last 50 years are a credit to the avid attention and painstaking labors undertaken by the many pathologists, surgeons, radiotherapists, and medical oncologists involved in the diagnosis and care of these patients. Hodgkin's lymphoma has been utilized as a paradigm of what can be done therapeutically to alter the natural history of neoplastic disease. The differences in clinical response, disease-free survival, and overall survival that have occurred clearly illustrate this fact. Therapeutically, this has meant the gradual evolution of technology and practice to encompass the successful treatment of advanced disease. The development of basic radiation therapy principles (dose response to radiation, treatment of contiguous lymph node areas, and appropriate treatment port design) has given the radiation oncologist effective tools with which to work, resulting in greater predictability as to outcome and the potential for curative treatment in many patients with Stage I–III disease. The development of curative intensive polychemotherapy lagged somewhat behind that of radiation therapy. However, in the 1960s, through the concurrent pioneering work of many investigators, inroads were made into the treatment of patients with pathologically advanced disease who had previously been poorly responsive to radiation.

Presentation of Disease

The histopathological description of the Hodgkin's lymphomas is illustrated in Table 1. The predominant form of Hodgkin's lym-

Table 1
Histopathology of the Hodgkin's Lymphomas

	Patients	*LP*	*NS*	*MC*	*LD*	*B-Symptoms*	*Male : Female*
Jackson* (before 1944)	112	23%	53%		24%		
Lukes** (1942–66)	394	16%	38%	25%	21%	42%	all males
Keller (1956–66)	179	5%	52%	37%	6%	39%	6:4
Kaplan*** (1961–77)	1,225	6%	67%	18%	2%	34%	6:4
Bergsagel*** (1968–77)	780	9%	61%	26%	3%	32%	6:4
TOTALS:***	2,561	8%	60%	23%	6%		

LP: lymphocyte predominant
NS: nodular sclerosing
MC: mixed cellularity
LD: lymphocyte depletion
*Histological subtypes from studies of Jackson were translated as follows: paragranuloma = LP, granuloma = NS + MC, and sarcoma = LD.
**Histological subtypes from the studies of Lukes et al. were translated as follows: lymphocyte/histiocyte nodular and diffuse = LP, diffuse fibrosis and reticular = LD.
***Does not include cases classified as undifferentiated.

phoma seen is the nodular sclerosing variant representing a cumulative 60% of the total. The lymphocyte predominant and depleted variants both account for less than 10% of the grouping, with the mixed cellularity subtype occupying an intermediate position at 23% of the Hodgkin's lymphomas. Studies from before the mid-1960s illustrated in Table 1 are translated when possible into the current Rye Conference terminology for purposes of comparison with the newer studies. The overall histological trends seem unchanged with the nodular sclerosing and mixed cellularity subtypes predominant throughout.

The age of disease onset has unique trends for each of the histological subgroups. Nodular sclerosis subtype incidence peaks in the second and third decades of life, with a mild female to male dominance. The frequency rapidly tapers such that by the fourth decade it is no more common than the mixed cellularity subtype. The latter subtype peaks in incidence in the third and fourth decades. Lymphocyte-predominant and lymphocyte-depleted histologies have more even distributions; lymphocyte-depleted histology occurs more frequently in older patients. The net result is unlike non-Hodgkin's lymphomas and shows a bimodal character. The overall median age is young (30) with an overwhelming predominance of nodular sclerosis as subtype in that age group. However, the older population is more evenly split between mixed cellularity and nodular sclerosing subtypes with a concurrent mild increase in the incidence of lymphocyte-depleted histology. These factors imply that the elderly population is more likely to have advanced and symptomatic disease. The rest of the histological subtypes (other than nodular sclerosing) account for an overall 60:40 male predominance of the disease. Constitutional (B) symptoms are present overall in 35% of the compiled series.

Stage at presentation for each of the Hodgkin's lymphomas is reflected in the composite data of Table 2. A minority of patients present with advanced disease. Fully 61% present with Stage I or II disease after pathological staging, a figure much greater than either nodular or diffuse non-Hodgkin's lymphomas. Pathological staging in Hodgkin's lymphoma leads to the diagnosis of more advanced disease. However, because of the predominance of Stage I and II disease, upstaging is less common than in most of the non-Hodgkin's lymphomas. Stage at presentation is not entirely independent of histology. Nodular sclerosing subtype (representing 60% of all disease) most commonly presents with Stage I or II disease. Mixed cellularity and especially lymphocyte-depleted histologies more commonly present with an advanced stage and symptomatic disease. Hodgkin's lymphoma of any stage presenting with constitutional symptoms is associated with more extensive and aggressive disease. This is often difficult to document pathologically. In addition, patients presenting with bulky Stage II mediastinal disease (greater than one-third the chest diameter) or Stage III_2 disease involving the lower paraaortic abdominal lymph nodes represent anatomical subsets of disease more difficult to treat.

Since the classical work of Rosenberg and Kaplan, systematic evaluation has established the role of contiguous spread of Hodgkin's

Table 2
Hodgkin's Lymphomas—Presentation by Stage

	Patients	*I*	*II*	*III*	*IV*
*Lukes (1942–66)	112	38%	34%	28%	
Keller (1956–66)	179	63%		37%	
Kaplan (1961–77)	1,225	11%	47%	31%	11%
Bergsagel (1968–77)	780	19%	40%	26%	15%

*Staging adapted from Stages I–III of Peters.

disease. Pattern of disease presentation, relapse, and sites of disease at autopsy bear this out. To Kaplan, contiguity in Hodgkin's lymphoma refers to "the existence of direct connections between pairs of lymph node chains by way of one or more lymphatic channels which do not have to pass through and be filtered by lymph node barriers"—implying lymphatic dissemination of disease. Analysis of this hypothesis shows contiguity to be present greater than 90% of the time when node-bearing areas are evaluated for mode of spread. In Hodgkin's lymphoma, there is a high concordance role between subdiaphragmatic disease in the paraaortic nodes in patients who were only clinically staged I or II with supraclavicular/mediastinal nodes.

Initial sites of disease presentation have been evaluated in staging studies as illustrated in Table 3. This particular collection of 272 patients from the Stanford series is illustrative. There is a high incidence

Table 3
Sites of Presentation of Hodgkin's Lymphoma

Stage I–III Nodal Presentation in 272 Patients	
Above Diaphragm	*% Involvement*
Left supraclavicular	73
Right supraclavicular	65
Mediastinum	63
Left and right axillary	26
Left and right hilar	22
Infraclavicular	9
Internal mammary	4
Epitrochlear	1
Waldeyer's ring	1
Below Diaphragm	
Spleen	36
Celiac/periaortics	33
Splenic hilar	13
Iliacs	13
Inguinal	9
Mesenterics	1
Extralymphatic Presentation	
	% Involvement
Pulmonary	9
Bone	7
Bone marrow	3
Liver	3
Pericardium	2
Skin	2

of supraclavicular node and mediastinal adenopathy. The incidence of mesenteric, head and neck, and epitrochlear adenopathy is much lower than that seen in the non-Hodgkin's lymphomas. Besides the striking lower incidence of mesenteric node involvement, there is a lower overall incidence of abdominal node involvement. Much of this can be attributed to the predominant presentation of the nodular sclerosis subtype with supradiaphragmatic pathology and to the lower incidence of Stage III and IV disease. Spleen and celiac nodes are the most commonly involved intraabdominal lymphatics. There is also a low incidence of Stage IV extralymphatic presentations, with a different trend from non-Hodgkin's lymphoma in presenting sites. Pulmonary parenchymal involvement is the most common Stage IV site of disease, followed by bone and bone marrow (seen only in 3% of patients in this particular series). In contrast with the non-Hodgkin's lymphomas, gastrointestinal tract (excluding liver) and primary central nervous system presentations were almost never seen.

Anatomical sites at autopsy are well described in numerous older studies, emphasizing the transition to increasing foci of lymphatic and extralymphatic disease. Sites seldom suspected at presentation are commonly involved at autopsy with bone marrow, bone, and liver being most frequent. A recent review of the autopsy experience over the past 25 years at the National Cancer Institute emphasizes the role of vascular invasion as a precursor to extranodal involvement—involving some 43% of the 143 patients autopsied. Two particular trends stood out. There was a reduction in the extent of disease in patients treated in the modern era of radiation and chemotherapy after 1965, particularly in lymphatic sites. Secondly, an altered histological form of disease ("treatment-altered Hodgkin's") was present in many of the patients, especially those treated after 1965.

Clinical Course

The natural history of Hodgkin's lymphoma as it has evolved from palliative therapy to our present day standards of care has received elegant appraisal by various authors. Prior to the onset of effective therapeutic modalities, the survival curve for Hodgkin's lymphoma was almost first order with a constant predictable failure and death rate. The dramatic impact of therapy on survival is illustrated by the cumulative data presented in Table 4, drawn from the indicated sources. As can be inferred, the initial impact on survival occurred with the successful use of tumor-sterilizing doses of kilovoltage ra-

Table 4
Survival of Patients with Hodgkin's Disease–Natural History

	5-Year Survival	*10-Year Survival*
Composite data from pretreatment era*	8%	1%
Peters (before 1950)	36%	23%
Lukes (1942–66)	40%	22%
Keller (1956–66)	57%	—
Kaplan (1961–77)	81%	67%
Bergsagel (1968–77)	80%	70%

*From Kaplan, H.S.: *Hodgkin's Disease* (2nd ed.). Cambridge, Massachusetts, Harvard University Press, 1980.

diation. The first long-term, disease-free survivors came from that group. They were followed in turn by patients treated by more effective dosages and modalities of radiation from the linear accelerator in the 1960s. Finally, the last studies reflect the influence of polymodality chemotherapy in the latter 1960s and recent decade of the 1970s with its impact on the patients with advanced refractory disease.

In the Hodgkin's lymphomas, the course of disease is governed by stage (anatomical extent of disease) more than by histopathological subtype, though these are not truly independent variables. The influence of modern therapy has been felt most acutely in advanced disease. Table 5 illustrates some of these data. Five- and ten-year survivals show their greatest improvements as a function of advancing stage. Specific problems for treatment planning and outcome are engendered by various combinations of disease at presentation. Stage II disease with a massively enlarged mediastinum, Stage $IIIA_2$ disease with lower abdominal nodal involvement, any stage with extralymphatic contiguity, or any stage with the presence of B symptoms are examples of such problems. These are detailed in the therapeutics section.

Table 5
Hodgkin's Disease—Survival by Stage

	I		II		III		IV	
	5-Yr	*10-Yr*	*5-Yr*	*10-Yr*	*5-Yr*	*10-Yr*	*5-Yr*	*10-Yr*
*Lukes (1942–66)	70%	47%	30%	10%	13%	2%		
Keller (1956–66)	90%		65%		40%		20%	
Kaplan (1961–77)	90%	79%	88%	74%	74%	57%	57%	40%

*Staging from Peters with three stage system, Stage III disease correlates most closely with Stage III and IV disease by current Ann Arbor staging classification.

Rebiopsy studies of recurrent disease in Hodgkin's lymphoma show little to no progression to more aggressive histology (LD) in patients with nodular sclerosis subtype, but rates of progression up to 25% in mixed cellularity. In the small subgroup of patients with lymphocyte predominant histology with relapse, rebiopsy will show histological progression greater than 60% of the time to less favorable forms, consistent with an evolutionary view of pathological progression of the disease.

The spread and relapse of Hodgkin's lymphoma to both lymphatic and extralymphatic sites has been described. The frequency and nature of noncontiguous relapse patterns are between 20–25%. Noncontiguous spread correlates, as does survival with evidence of less favorable histological subtypes (mixed cellularity and lymphocyte depletion), with vascular invasion, particularly in those patients with constitutional symptoms. Studies have equated the presence of vascular invasion and splenic lymphoma with evidence of hematogenous spread and a subsequent propensity for bone marrow involvement.

Factors most predictive of outcome in the Hodgkin's lymphomas include advanced stage and histopathology, as well as the presence of constitutional symptoms. Mixed cellularity and lymphocyte depletion pathologies are commonly associated with a more advanced stage and a greater frequency of B symptoms. A variety of additional factors suggest a less favorable outcome including age, initial intraabdominal presentation, splenic involvement, bone marrow disease, and bulky mediastinal involvement. A high incidence of subsequent treatment failure of an extranodal variety can be predicted.

As the survival data clearly indicate, there has been a dramatic change in the outcome of the Hodgkin's lymphomas. Their natural history after treatment is unique from that of some non-Hodgkin's lymphomas, affording an opportunity to provide significant prolongation of survival.

Non-Hodgkin's Lymphomas

The historical background to the non-Hodgkin's lymphomas reaches back into the 1800s. Previously grouped with Hodgkin's lymphoma, it was during the early 1900s that histological criteria were formulated, allowing lymphosarcoma, reticulum cell sarcoma, and follicular sarcomas (precursors of our modern histologic subtypes) to be recognized as distinct pathological entities, separate from Hodgkin's lymphoma. Unfortunately, the early natural history studies by Gall and Rosenberg utilizing these histological terms do not readily translate into present schemas. Lack of reproducibility together with heterogeneity within groups led to further classification systems which we now employ more successfully. Although histopathological schemas have been a problem, it has been their development and refinement that has led the way to understanding what is known about the natural history of non-Hodgkin's lymphoma. Other predictors are important (anatomic stage, age, sex, B-symptoms, etc.); however, it is histopathological subtype that is the driving force behind the course of the non-Hodgkin's diseases.

Therapeutically, the natural history of non-Hodgkin's lymphomas began to change with the advent of radiotherapy. Orthovoltage therapy first caused responses and palliation of symptoms. Gradual evolution in the technology and application of radiation physics has led to the understanding of what radiation therapy can do to alter outcome in these diseases:

(1) There is a definite dose response effect of radiation on lymphatic malignancies.
(2) When treatment is of curative intent, there is a need for concurrent radiation of uninvolved as well as involved lymphatic tissue.
(3) In anatomically limited disease, radiotherapy is potentially curative.

Borrowing from the experience with Hodgkin's lymphomas, the assessment in the 1950s that a small fraction of these patients may be potentially curable brought about the first major historical impact on the natural history of the non-Hodgkin's lymphomas. As these concepts of radiotherapy developed, data have accumulated, allowing relatively accurate prediction of who will and will not benefit from radiotherapy.

Since the introduction of nitrogen mustard in the 1940s, there has been a gradual inroad of chemotherapy on the natural history of some of the non-Hodgkin's lymphomas. Modest and sporadic treatment with a limited number of agents in the early years afforded palliation of symptoms and partial responses, primarily in the indolent lymphomas. With the advent of aggressive polychemotherapy programs in the last 15 years has come the first evidence for major alterations of the natural history of the more aggressive lymphomas.

Non-Hodgkin's Lymphoma: Indolent Histologies

The first group of lymphomas to be considered include the indolent histology lymphomas. Cell types include:

Nodular poorly differentiated lymphocytic	(NPDL or follicular small cleaved cell)
Nodular mixed	(NML or follicular mixed small cleaved and large cell lymphoma)
Diffuse poorly differentiated lymphocytic	(DPDL or diffuse small cleaved cell)
Well-differentiated lymphocytic lymphoma	(WDLL or diffuse small lymphocytes)

These cell types share a number of common synonyms describing their overall character and clinical course: indolent, favorable histology, low grade, and relapsing malignancies. (*Note:* Nodular histiocytic cell type is considered less favorable and not grouped with the other two nodular subtypes. DPDL and WDLL lymphomas are grouped prognostically with the indolent lymphomas because of their initial stage of presentation, response to therapy, and chronic pattern of relapse.) Most studies of pathology or natural history subdivide by nodular and diffuse histologies. The designations used here (indolent and aggressive lymphomas) encompass aspects of both. Therefore, in subsequent discussions it must be remembered that the indolent lymphomas have both nodular and diffuse subtypes.

Presentation of Disease

Indolent lymphomas comprise about 50% of all non-Hodgkin's lymphomas. Table 6 represents a composite of several histopathological studies that deal with the issue of histopathological frequency based on the Rappaport classification. NPDL is the most common nodular variant, representing 21.8% of the non-Hodgkin's lymphomas, followed by NML and NHL at 16.1% and 4.9%, respectively. As can be seen from the data, there is intergroup consistency both in terms of the overall percentage of non-Hodgkin's lymphomas and in regard to the various histological nodular subytpes. The variance in frequency of NML is due to the variation in the proportion of small and large cells which are used to define the entities by differing histopathologists.

Table 6
Histopathological Breakdown of Non-Hodgkin's Lymphomas by Historical Studies*

	Rappaport** (before 1956)	Patchefsky (1950–71)	Jones (1950–71)	Goffinet (1971–76)	Anderson (1953–75)	TOTAL
Total Patient #	235	293	405	423	473	1594
Nodular Histology	100%	44%	43%	48%	38%	43.0%
NWDL	10%	1%	1%	—	—	0.6%
NPDL	45%	22%	17%	30%	19%	21.8%
NML	35%	18%	18%	13%	16%	16.1%
NHL	10%	3%	7%	5%	3%	4.9%
Diffuse Histology		56%	57%	52%	62%	57.0%
WDLL		2%	2%	3%	8%	4.8%
DPDL		15%	11%	13%	14%	13.0%
DML		10%	11%	4%	7%	7.7%
DHL		26%	29%	29%	19%	25.4%
DUL		3%	4%	3%	6%	3.8%
Burkitt's		—	—	—	8%	2.4%

*Figure for all patients (includes both diffuse and nodular histologies).
**Patients from this group not included in total patient numbers.

Of note is that WDLL and DPDL together only account for about 18% of all non-Hodgkin's lymphomas.

Of particular importance is the fact that between 10–15% of patients who undergo complete pathological staging have more than one histological subtype present synchronously, either within a given nodal site (so-called composite lymphoma) or in differing nodal sites. A retrospective analysis of one large group of these patients shows that the survival of patients with more than one histological type of non-Hodgkin's lymphoma is intermediate between that expected for either subtype. This variable of histological presentation may account for difficulty in interpretation of clinical responses.

Indolent lymphomas usually present with advanced stages of disease. In fact, it is this curious combination of advanced stage at diagnosis with prolonged survival that provides the interesting paradox surrounding these lymphomas. Though indolent in nature and favorable in regard to overall survival, they are essentially incurable, with a continued late relapse rate. Clinical and pathological staging studies of these entities have been extensive. The results shown here (Table 7) represent a composite of previously noted studies. Systematic staging procedures were not done before the 1960s in a fashion that we currently accept as complete.

Table 7
Clinical and Pathological Staging of Non-Hodgkin's Lymphomas

	Patchefsky* (1950–71)	Jones** (1960–71)	Goffinet (1971–76)	Anderson (1953–75)
Nodular Histology				
Pathological Stage				
I	}39	10.7	8.2	6.2
II		21.9	13.1	9.6
III	}61	33.7	29.1	34.8
IV		33.7	49.5	49.4
Diffuse Histology				
Pathological Stage				
I	}37	13.6	16.1	7.6
II		26.9	32.2	14.9
III	}63	16.7	12.0	24.3
IV		42.7	39.6	53.7

*Clinical staging only.
**Clinical and pathological staging.

Staging studies from 1960 or earlier have to be interpreted carefully. These observations are possible:

(1) Indolent (or lymphocytic) lymphomas usually present with Stage III or IV disease.
(2) The application of more systematic staging procedures in the recent years has led to the diagnosis of more advanced Stage III and IV disease from 60–65% to greater than 80% with rigorous staging criteria.

For the indolent non-Hodgkin's lymphomas, the mean age of onset is 45–50 (except for DPDL) with the peak incidence in the sixth decade of life. Although childhood and early adult indolent non-Hodgkin's lymphomas do occur, the greatest number of non-Hodgkin's lymphomas prevalent in early life are aggressive in character and diffuse in histology. Similarly, though a male predominance has been cited in non-Hodgkin's lymphoma, the difference is not marked. A modest male predilection occurs only in the more aggressive diffuse histological subtypes.

Disease presentation can be discussed on three levels: (1) pattern of spread at presentation (contiguity), (2) lymphatic sites of involvement, and (3) extranodal sites of involvement. A totally accurate assessment of presenting sites is only possible if meticulous staging procedures have been undertaken. These include appropriate biopsies and laparotomy with splenectomy. As has been documented numerous times, studies based on clinical assessment alone are not accurate for this purpose. However, anatomical staging may not always be required for treatment decisions.

Since the demonstration by Kaplan and Rosenberg that Hodgkin's lymphoma presents and spreads in lymphatic tissue by a contiguous nonrandom fashion, these same principles of presentation have been applied to non-Hodgkin's lymphoma. Contiguous spread of disease is defined as that occurring to adjacent lymph node-bearing areas which are directly connected by lymph node channels. From the previous work with Hodgkin's lymphoma, this has implied contiguity between paraaortic and supraclavicular nodes via the thoracic duct (with or without concurrent mediastinal involvement). In patients with non-Hodgkin's lymphoma who present with limited pathological Stage II or III disease, there is contiguity of spread in 87% and 71%, respectively, by stage including all histological types. Contiguity, however, decreases to 65% in indolent disease while remaining extremely high at 95% in aggressive subtypes. Contiguity ranges from a low of 57% in patients with Waldeyer's ring involvement to over 90% in patients with paraaortic and supraclavicular node adenopathy.

Experience with sites of disease at presentation has been gained through staging studies. However, extensive data on sites of disease and pattern of spread at relapse have been more difficult to gather. Table 8 summarizes data by site for initial sites of presentation in Stages I–III and for extranodal Stage IV disease, as seen in the collective Stanford experience from 1971–76. A variety of less frequently involved sites, including testis, central nervous system, epidural space, breast, and pericardium have been documented. Though given collectively in Table 8, a substantial difference exists in site of involvement between histologies. Indolent histologies involve mesenteric, paraaortic, and splenic hilar nodes between 61–71% of the time compared with a range of 25–42% in the more aggressive diffuse histologies. Bone marrow involvement at the time of initial diagnosis in indolent lymphomas varies from a low of 35–40% to a high of 76% in pathologically staged subtypes. Marrow involvement is a common rather than unusual occurrence. Involvement at presentation for aggressive pathologies is between 10–15%.

Autopsy and rebiopsy studies show a gradual transition towards extralymphatic involvement and less well-differentiated histologies with the progress of the disease. In older studies, such as reported by Rappaport on 76 autopsies of follicular lymphoma, a substantial percentage of extralymphatic sites were involved: bone marrow (47%), kidney (35%), lungs (29%), and gastrointestinal tract (29%). Later

Table 8
Sites of Presentation of Non-Hodgkin's Lymphoma

Stage I–III Nodal Presentation in 144 Patients Including Spleen–All Histological Types	
Below Diaphragm	*% Involvement*
Iliac/Femoral Nodes	59
Paraaortics	50
Spleen	42
Mesenterics	41
Above Diaphragm	
Left Cervical	55
Left Supraclavicular	49
Right Cervical	46
Right Supraclavicular	37
Axillary	29
Mediastinum	24
Waldeyer's Ring	10
Stage IV Extranodal Disease in 423 Patients at Presentation All Histological Types	
	% Involvement
Bone Marrow	32
Liver	8
Skin	6
Lung	6
Bone	4
Small Bowel	4
Pleural Effusion	3
Stomach	3
CNS	2

autopsy studies undertaken in all histologies after the onset of aggressive chemotherapy and radiotherapy programs show a higher incidence of liver, renal, gastrointestinal, and central nervous system involvement.

Clinical Course

The natural history of untreated indolent non-Hodgkin's lymphoma has been a subject of debate and is the object of continued clinical investigation. There are currently ongoing clinical trials looking specifically at the issue of no initial therapy in the indolent lymphomas versus more aggressive treatment with single agent and polymodality therapy.

In a study by Portlock, there were 44 patients with indolent histologies who were unwilling or unable to be included in prospective group protocols involving drugs or radiotherapy. This special group of patients was followed until such time as their disease showed symptoms that needed treatment. Six of those 44 patients underwent spontaneous remission, of which four were prolonged without therapy. Median survivals were not notably different in these patients from historical controls who had received earlier treatments on protocol.

Potential hazards of such an approach include the evolution of silent disease, psychological burden of untreated disease, and the advancement of disease to a greater stage or site that might adversely affect survival and response rate. The rationale for such an approach is based on the supposition that the natural history of indolent lymphomas includes a certain percentage of these tumors that will evolve into more aggressive diffuse histologies that might be curable with present day therapy. Early therapy may negatively prejudice the response of the more aggressive lymphoma. In addition, treatment-related morbidity may be worse than no treatment in an otherwise asymptomatic individual. When all patients are rebiopsied prospectively the rate of such histological conversion approached 30% in small studies. Given the relatively poor outcome of patients with histological progression who are pretreated, hypothetical considerations for less aggressive initial management may help define the natural history of these indolent subtypes and best alternatives for therapy. Currently there are ongoing prospective studies underway that seek to answer these questions directly.

The effect on the natural history of any disease can be reflected in part by changing survival data in the face of contemporary treatment modalities. A comparison of survival by histologic subtype and periods of diagnosis is shown in Table 9.

Causes of death in indolent lymphoma are related to persistence of disease. From the autopsy series of Rappaport in the 1950s, death related to the underlying lymphoma occurred in 67 of 76 patients (88%). Four of the 67 disease-related deaths were treatment-induced. Overall sites of organ involvement at autopsy were primarily nodal, with bone marrow, liver, lung, and kidney the only extralymphatic sites with greater than 10% involvement. Seventy-two of the 76 patients had some evidence of lymphoma at autopsy. In a later series from the past decade, cause of death is notably altered by the prior use of radiotherapy or chemotherapy in the treatment of non-Hodgkin's lymphoma. In patients who are intensively pretreated, there is a combination of treatment-induced toxicity and advanced extranodal disease.

As the survival data suggest, there has been, at most, a modest improvement in the overall duration of survival in the indolent lymphomas. There has been no demonstration yet that cure is an attainable goal in these subtypes. The problems of constant relapse are well demonstrated by the actuarial data summarized in Chapter 6, *Chemotherapy of the Lymphomas*. The modest improvement in survival does not seem to be due to changes in pathological subtypes, stage of presentation, or other selection factors. It may correlate with the onset of new treatment modalities and better methods of patient support. Whether additional improvements in chemotherapy or radiotherapy will provide a substantial improvement or the potential for long-term, disease-free survival remains to be seen.

In summary, the natural history of the indolent lymphomas is that of a chronic, relapsing and incurable disease whose overall course can only be palliated.

Non-Hodgkin's Lymphoma: Aggressive Histologies

The group of aggressive histology lymphomas to be considered includes several of Rappaport's diffuse lymphomas. Cell types include:

Nodular histiocytic	(NHL, follicular large cell)
Diffuse mixed	(DML, diffuse mixed small cleaved and large cell)
Diffuse histiocytic	(DHL, diffuse large cell or diffuse large cell immunoblastic)
Diffuse undifferentiated	(DUL, non-Burkitt's and Burkitt's)
Lymphoblastic	(Lymphoblastic)

The "diffuse" designation has remained a part of the Working Formulation classification indicated on the right. Controversy surrounds the Rappaport designation of diffuse histiocytic and undifferentiated lymphomas. Data accumulated in Tables 6–10 to describe the natural history of DHL and DUL cannot be translated easily into the terminology of the Working Formulation as there are now subdivisions of DHL.

Presentation of Disease

Aggressive lymphomas comprise between 45–50% of all the non-Hodgkin's lymphomas. Reference to Table 6 shows composite data for the major histopathological subtypes. The predominant Rappaport

Table 9
Non-Hodgkin's Lymphomas

	Median Survival in Months Rappaport (Before 1956)	Patchefsky (1950–71)	Jones (1950–71)	Anderson (1953–73)	Anderson (1968–73)
Nodular Histology					
NWDL	50	NR*	NR	—	—
NPDL	50	72	105	78	108
NML	36	34	96	55	100
NHL	36	12	44	29	20
	Gall (Before 1940)				
Diffuse Histology					
WDLL	28	NR	NR	67	84
DPDL	7	30	23	20	24
DML	—	12	22	20	36
DHL	12	12	13	10	10
DUL	—	10	8	10	18
Burkitt's	—	—	—	10	12

NR* median survival not reached.

category is DHL constituting about 25% of all non-Hodgkin's lymphomas. The rest of the aggressive subtypes constitute less than 10% each. Of note is the high incidence of Burkitt's-type lymphomas in the latter study group. This is reflective of referral patterns to that institution and not of an overall change in the natural occurrence of the disease. There appears to be little change with time in the incidence of the various subtypes. Considering the difficulty with pathological diagnosis, concordance rates are remarkably consistent. The mild

Table 10
Influence of Multiple Agent Chemotherapy on Survival in Aggressive Non-Hodgkin's Lymphoma

	Survival Before 1968		*Survival After 1968*	
Pathological Subtype	Median Survival (Months)	% 5-Yr. Survival	Median Survival (Months)	% 5-Yr. Survival
WDLL	67	45	88	65
DPDL	20	20	24	25
DML	20	10	36	48
DHL	10	12	10	35
DUL	10	0	18	15
Burkitt's	8	30	8	50

downward trend in DHL is a reflection of efforts at reclassification of the heterogeneous group of large cell lymphomas. It should be remembered, parenthetically, that 10–15% of patients classified as having aggressive lymphomas may also have concurrent indolent disease initially present in nodal sites.

As with indolent subtypes, the application of systematic staging procedures has shown an increased incidence of advanced pathological stages in aggressive lymphomas. The patterns of presentation, however, are unique from the indolent lymphomas (see Table 7). There are greater numbers of histological subtypes with pathologically less advanced (Stages I and II) disease, ranging from a low of 22.5% in the National Cancer Institute review by Anderson to a high of 48.3% in the Stanford series of Goffinet. Consequently there are fewer patients with Stage III and Stage IV disease. Of interest is the variation by specific histological subtype. DWDL and DPDL (diffuse but indolent pathologies) present with advanced (Stage III or IV pathologic) disease 95% and 78% of the time, respectively. The aggressive lymphoma categories account for a much lower percentage of advanced disease. Fully 37% of the more aggressive histologies of this group present as pathological Stage I or Stage II disease (see Table 7).

Although median age does not differ appreciably on a collective basis, several groups have distinct trends. DPDL (indolent subtype) and DUL peak in the fourth decade with a median age of 34. Burkitt's-type lymphoma has a median age of 8, reported in the most recent accumulated studies from the National Cancer Institute.

Earlier in this chapter, disease presentation in regard to site of involvement was discussed for both major categories of lymphomas. Contiguity of spread in the aggressive lymphomas (approaching 95%) is more reminiscent of Hodgkin's lymphoma than the indolent diseases. Breakdown of contiguity occurs only between paraaortic and supraclavicular node involvement. Eighty to 85% of these nodal areas are contiguous in the aggressive pathologies, compared with nearly 100% in the indolent subtypes.

There is a lower incidence of mesenteric and subdiaphragmatic node, spleen, and liver involvement in the aggressive lymphomas. Though mediastinal adenopathy is common in the Hodgkin's lymphomas, its appearance in non-Hodgkin's lymphoma is less frequent. At presentation, mediastinal nodes are involved in the non-Hodgkin's diseases between 20–30% of the time according to combined data from the major sources.

The incidence and sites of extranodal involvement in patients with

Stage IV disease on presentation is detailed in Table 8. Several important points need emphasis:

(1) Patients with aggressive lymphomas have a lower incidence of Stage IV disease at presentation.

(2) Excluding liver and bone marrow, 75–80% of the extranodal sites at presentation occur in aggressive histologies.

(3) The occurrence of primary (Stage IE, pathologic) extranodal non-Hodgkin's lymphoma without other sites of disease is more common to aggressive than to indolent pathologies. In one representative series, 72% (28/39 patients) were of aggressive pathological subtypes. Median age was 55 with an equal sex ratio. The most common sites of initial involvement by aggressive lymphoma were the gastrointestinal tract and head and neck (Waldeyer's ring and sinuses) in 24/39 patients, or 59% of the total group. Less commonly involved primary sites included bone 13%, testes and thyroid 8%, and breast and CNS 6%. Survival again was related to histopathological subtype, extent, and site of disease. Relapse sites in these presentations are often noncontiguous (33%).

Autopsy studies looking at the site of involvement in the aggressive lymphomas revealed involvement of extranodal sites beyond those which normally are involved at presentation. In a recent review of autopsy data from patients with primarily aggressive histologies, the more frequent sites of involvement were: lungs (29%), bone marrow (26%), liver (24%), and kidney (23%) with less frequent involvement of the gastrointestinal tract (20%), spleen (19%), central nervous system (13%), and cardiovascular system (13%).

Clinical Course

The natural history of most aggressive lymphomas (untreated) is not controversial. The survival of untreated disease has been limited.

Table 9 reflects the natural history of the various histologies up to and including the beginning of the past decade. Trials of *radiotherapy or single agent chemotherapy* have proven of little use. There has been an insignificant impact on the survival of these diseases. Curative radiotherapy for localized pathological Stage I disease is the only notable exception. Although the dose response data of radiation therapy on aggressive lymphomas show higher local relapse rates than in indolent disease, it has been used successfully in true Stage I disease.

The use of single agent chemotherapy in the more aggressive histologies does not improve survival.

What has occurred in the interim is the advent of polymodality chemotherapy programs (sometimes in combination with radiation) with their impact on the natural history of these diseases. This can be measured by three parameters: complete response to therapy, median survival, and percentage of long-term, disease-free survivors. In indolent histologies, such an analysis is difficult to make because of the constant relapse/failure rate even after complete remission. The aggressive diffuse histologies are in stark contrast. Their relapse rate is very low after remissions of greater than 2 years. Based on the analysis of data before and after 1968 at the National Cancer Institute, there is a gradually improving trend in the survival of the aggressive lymphomas, particularly of pathological Stage III and Stage IV disease. Table 10 is extrapolated from that data (indolent pathology DPDL and WDLL are included for purposes of comparison). A number of important observations can be made:

(1) The major impact of prolonged survival has occurred in pathologically advanced (Stages III and IV) disease with the onset of polychemotherapy.
(2) Although overall median survival has begun to show improvement, there are still major groups of refractory disease that keep median survival relatively low. This has been detailed in the chapter on the treatment of disease.
(3) There is an increase in prolonged, disease-free survival among aggressive subtypes in DML, DHL, Burkitt's, and to lesser degrees in DUL. Pathological Stage III and Stage IV diseases within these subgroups is where the natural history is most significantly altered. The subgroups WDLL and DPDL (grouped with the indolent pathologies) have shown less alteration in median survival or long-term, disease-free survival than the aggressive subgroups.

Whether these improvements in complete response, etc. translate into radical alteration of the natural history (potential for cure) is dependent on ongoing prospective trials with long-term follow-up in well-designed clinical trials. Extensive discussion of the factors other than histopathology predicting positive treatment outcomes is beyond the scope of this discussion. In the aggressive lymphomas, other important factors predictive of outcome include the presence of B symptoms, bone marrow involvement, advanced stage of disease, and large intraabdominal masses.

Causes of death in the aggressive lymphomas have changed as

have the patterns of treatment. Causes of death frequently relate to acute and cumulative toxicity of treatment as well as advancing disease. From a recent autopsy series examining end-stage lymphoma patients, 104 of 119 patients had evidence of lymphoma at the time of death. Thirty-two patients of 119 patients died of infection, with 20 of those 32 patients being granulocytopenic due to therapy at the time. Twenty-nine patients died of respiratory insufficiency apart from pneumonia, with diseased lung and pulmonary drug toxicity as the leading causes. Fourteen of 119 patients died of hemorrhage directly referrable to thrombocytopenia resulting from chemotherapy. The gastrointestinal tract, cardiovascular system, and central nervous system were involved to a greater degree than in the previously published series. A burgeoning literature in recent years shows an increased incidence of leukemia and other secondary hematological malignancies in patients successfully treated for their prior lymphoma.

The character and natural history of the aggressive non-Hodgkin's lymphomas are unique from those of the indolent variety. It appears that we may be in the process of seeing a true alteration in treatment responsiveness that translates to the measure of altered natural history—biologically meaningful increased survival. Prolonged observation and well-designed clinical trials will aid in confirming that impression.

Selected Reading

Hodgkin's Lymphoma

Bergsagel, D.E., Alison, R.G., Bean, H.A., et al.: Results of treating Hodgkin's disease without a policy of laparotomy staging. *Cancer Treatment Rep.* 66(4):717–731, 1982.

Grogan, T.M., Berard, C.W., Steinhorn, S.C., et al.: Changing patterns of Hodgkin's disease at autopsy: A 25-year experience at the National Cancer Institute, 1953–78. *Cancer Treatment Rep.* 66(4):653–665, 1982.

Jackson, H., Parker, F.: Hodgkin's disease. II. Pathology. *N. Engl. J. Med.* 231(2):35–44, 1944.

Kaplan, H.S.: *Hodgkin's Disease* (2nd ed.). Cambridge, Massachusetts, Harvard University Press, 1980.

Kaplan, H.S., Dorfman, R.F., Nelsen, T.S., et al.: Staging, laparotomy and splenectomy in Hodgkin's disease: Analysis of indicators and patterns of involvement in 285 consecutive, unselected patients. *National Cancer Institute Monograph* 36:291–301, 1973.

Keller, A.R., Kaplan, H.S., Lukes, R.J., et al.: Correlation of histopathology with other prognostic indicators in Hodgkin's disease. *Cancer* 22(3):487–499, 1968.

Lukes, R.J., Butler, J.J., Hicks, E.B.: Natural history of Hodgkin's disease as related to its pathologic picture. *Cancer* 19(3):317–344, 1966.

Peters, M.V.: A study of survivals in Hodgkin's disease treated radiologically. *Am. J. Roentgenol.* 63:299–311, 1950.

Rosenberg, S.A., Kaplan, H.S.: Evidence for an orderly progression in the spread of Hodgkin's disease. *Cancer Res.* 26:1225–1231, 1966.

Non-Hodgkin's Lymphoma

Anderson, T., Chabner, B.A., Young, R.C., et al.: Malignant lymphoma. I. The histology and staging of 473 patients at the National Cancer Institute. *Cancer* 50:2699–2707, 1982.

Anderson, T., DeVita, V.T., Simon, R.M., et al.: Malignant lymphoma. II. Prognostic factors and response to treatment of 473 patients at the National Cancer Institute. *Cancer* 50:2708–2721, 1982.

Fisher, R.I., Jones, R.B., DeVita, V.T., et al.: Natural history of malignant lymphomas with divergent histologies at staging evaluation. *Cancer* 47:2022–2025, 1981.

Fuks, Z., Glatstein, E., and Kaplan, H.S.: Patterns of presentation and relapse in the non-Hodgkin's lymphomata. *Br. J. Cancer* 31(Suppl. II):286–297, 1975.

Gall, E.A., Mahoney, T.B.: Malignant lymphoma. *Am. J. Pathol.* 18:381–429, 1941.

Goffinet, D.R., Warnke, R., Dunnick, N.R., et al.: Clinical and surgical (laparotomy) evaluation of patients with non-Hodgkin's lymphomas. *Cancer Treatment Rep.* 61:981–992, 1977.

Hubbard, S.M., Chabner, B.A., DeVita, V.T., et al.: Histologic progression in non-Hodgkin's lymphoma. *Blood* 59(2):258–264, 1982.

Jones, S.E., Fuks, Z., Bull, M., et al.: Non-Hodgkin's lymphomas. IV. Clinicopathologic correlation in 405 cases. *Cancer* 31:806–823, 1973.

Ostrow, S., Diggs, C.H., Sutherland, J., et al.: Causes of death in patients with non-Hodgkin's lymphoma. *Cancer* 48:779–782, 1981.

Patchefsky, A.S., Brodovsky, H.S., Menduke, H., et al.: Non-Hodgkin's lymphomas: A clinicopathologic study of 293 cases. *Cancer* 34:1173–1186, 1974.

Portlock, C.S., Rosenberg, S.A.: No initial therapy for stage III and IV non-Hodgkin's lymphomas of favorable histologic types. *Ann. Intern. Med.* 90:10–13, 1979.

Rappaport, H., Winten, W., Hicks, E.B.: Follicular lymphoma. *Cancer* 9(4):792–821, 1956.

Rosenberg, S.A., Diamond, H.D., Jaslowitz, B., et al.: Lymphosarcoma: A review of 1269 cases. *Medicine* 40:31–84, 1961.

Ruddens, R.A., Ross, M.G., Delellis, R.A.: Primary extranodal lymphoma. *Cancer* 42:406–416, 1978.

Straus, D.J., Flippa, D.A., Lieberman, P.H., et al.: The non-Hodgkin's lymphomas. I. A retrospective clinical and pathologic analysis of 499 cases diagnosed between 1958 and 1969. *Cancer* 51:101–109, 1983.

Warnke, R.A., Kim, H., Fuks, Z., et al.: The coexistence of nodular and diffuse patterns in nodular non-Hodgkin's lymphomas. *Cancer* 40:1229–1233, 1977.

Index